A Unique and Simplified Approach to
PHARMACY CALCULATIONS
For Healthcare Professionals

A Unique and Simplified Approach to
PHARMACY CALCULATIONS
For Healthcare Professionals

CHIDI OSUJI, Bsc.Pharm, M.Pharm
and
KINGSLEY OCHE, Bsc.Pharm, MSC

To order additional copies of this book, contact:
Xlibris
1-888-795-4274
www.Xlibris.com
Orders@Xlibris.com
760118

DEDICATION

To all students
who will find in this book
a reliable academic partner
in the sweet journey
into pharmacy
calculations.

To all institutions
who will employ this book
as an instrument for instructing students
in the science of pharmaceutical calculations.

To the loving memory of my late maternal grand parents:
Richard Ogonnaya & Agnes Obijialu Isuemenyiojoo,
whose tutelage cannot be easily forgotten.

To all who will in one way or the other
come in contact with
this piece.

How To Use This Book

As the name of this book implies, it presents pharmaceutical calculations in a very simple and unique manner such that it can be used, read and understood by all who venture into it despite background.

Each chapter begins with the objectives – what the chapter is prepared to impact to the reader. This is followed by a brief introduction of the concept of the chapter and some practice examples that are solved by the writer following some logical line of reasoning. 50 practice questions follow each chapter. Each chapter has one star question which is designed to incorporate the major concepts of the chapter. The answers to the practice questions, as well as the logical solution to the star questions, are presented at the end of each chapter.

In order to benefit maximally from this book, students should follow through the practice examples and the logic of their solutions before solving the practice questions.

Some students, most likely, have already mastered 'their own way' of solving proportion calculations. This is okay. It is, however, recommended that students put aside their own way of solving these kinds of calculations and have a second look at the way presented in this book. The way of this book may present yet a simplified approach that might clarify some calculation difficulties students might have.

It is recommended, also, that students solve the practice questions and the star questions on their own first before crosschecking the answers at the end of each chapter. In this way it will serve as a self-test to the students and also help in assessing students' understanding of the chapters. Chapter one is very essential in understanding the proportion concept of the entire book.

It should be noted that the explanations to the solutions in this book may be too annoyingly repetitive. Smart students may find this very boring, insulting and highly irritating. This was done on purpose. Its purpose is not to prove that all students are dull, but the book is designed such that no one is left behind in the trail of instruction, knowing fully well that many students join the medical profession career from different backgrounds and walks of life.

We wish all students a wonderful academic adventure in this piece. Be prepared to experience your 'aha!' moments as the exploration proceeds.

Chidi A. Osuji
Nolan Hill, Calgary, Alberta

Acknowledgments

For any intellectual product such as this book to see the light of the day, several people must have remotely or directly worked tirelessly and diligently to ensure the package emerges worthy of its name. For this reason I will not cease to express my gratitude to all the people who in one way or the other made this dream come true. Many of those people I will lack space to mention their names specifically. To all I say thank you, may you also meet assistance in times of your need.

To Kari Tannas, I say a big thank you for coming to my rescue and re-typing the manuscript when I needed your services most. I personally typed the manuscript of over 300 pages only to lose the work to a computer virus. At the point of despair, she stepped in and re-typed the work for me at an amazing speed and at a very subsidized rate. You are an angel!

My special gratitude goes to the team of content editors and reviewers who worked doggedly day and night to make sure this book meets its objective of being an academic resource to all professionals who handle medication. They read through, solved and re-confirmed calculations, detected and corrected minor technical errors and made some useful input that assisted in making the book come out more beautifully. I say a big thank you to Michael, Amandeep, Dr. Joseph, Adeola, Rev. Dr. Anthony, Laurence, Zubeda, Maher and Shehzaad. You are an awesome team.

My deep appreciation goes to the staff and management of Cambrooks College, Calgary, for the opportunity and confidence they placed on us to groom their students as pharmacy professionals. For making possible a serene academic environment where the harvest of intellectual talents is made possible, I will always express my gratitude to Prof. Faith-Michael Uzoka, Dr. Joseph Osuji, Emmanuel Aladi, Anthony Chima, Pamela, Joanne and Maureen. My special appreciation also goes to my past and present co-instructors (pharmacy) in the college, Dr. Chinyere, Islam, Dr. Syed and Kingsley for their excellent team spirit. My numerous students and other many erudite co-instructors are appreciated.

To my colleagues at Safeway/Sobeys where the dream for this book was initially hatched, I remain grateful. Special thanks to Shamoona, Laurence, Michael, Batul, Ayman, Robert, Vitalis, Chinenye, Andrea, Sangeeta, Joanne, David, Molly and Inder for their unalloyed support and encouragement.

To my previous academic project supervisors and assistant project supervisors back in the days at pharmacy faculty of the University of Nigeria, Nsukka, I say a big thank you. The academic light you kindled is not yet quenched. Special thank you to Prof. Vincent Okore, Prof. Sabinus Ofoefule and Prof. Kenneth Ofokansi.

Special thank you to Kingsley Oche, a pharmacist colleague and a friend for his major contribution of the appendix to the book, his review of the manuscript and pieces of advice as the writing progressed.

Special thanks to my family for all the support and encouragement throughout the chaotic process of the book writing, editing and publication. I am especially grateful to my wife Amarachi and our children Assumpta, Daniel, Michael, David and Emmanuel for providing the reasons to push hard and ahead. It is true that when a man is focused on a task, the immediate family feels the impact. Daniel and Assumpta even helped in the typesetting of the manuscript.

Finally, I can do nothing if not empowered by the source of real energy, the Grace, the Divine. I must appreciate that special Grace that quietly says 'yes, you can' even when the environment loudly shouts 'never!, impossible!!'.

Chidi Osuji

CONTRIBUTORS AND REVIEWERS

CONTRIBUTOR

Kingsley Oche, BPharm. MSc.

TECHNICAL EDITOR

Shehzaad Visram

MSc Mechanical Engineering,

BSc Chemistry & Biochemistry

TECHNICAL REVIEWERS

Mr. Michael Owolagba. BPharm

Zubeda Begum RPH M.Phill (Pharmaceutics)

Laurence Lee RPH

Amandeep Sekhon RPT

Dr. Joseph Osuji RN

Associate professor of Nursing

Mount Royal University

Adeola Babs-Mala (nee Fagbenro) B.Pharm

(University of Ibadan, Nigeria)

Rev. Dr. Anthony Osuji

Catholic Theologian

FOREWORD

Often times, pharmacists, allied professionals and students are faced with the difficult task of carrying out pharmaceutical calculations, which is an essential aspect of drug administration. More commonly, compounding calculations also present challenges to pharmacists, allied professionals and students. Compounding is both a science and art of ensuring that the patient receives appropriate amounts of ingredients in a medication mix based on a medical practitioner's prescription. The experiential knowledge of the pharmacist is brought to bear in the compounding process, which could make a lot of live-saving difference in patient recovery.

In this book, the authors have simply shared both factual and tacit experiential knowledge that presents a unique approach to pharmaceutical calculations, especially in the Canadian context. There is a fundamental recognition that most medical computations rely on the classical principles of proportions, which are mostly based on standardized units of medications that are composites of the pure drug substance(s) and inactive ingredients. The pharmacists must have the ability to interpret prescriptions to identify the active and other ingredients in order to carry out an appropriate compounding where the need arises.

The utility of this book lies in the authors' ability to greatly simplify pharmaceutical calculation concepts in a way that appeals to pharmacists, student-pharmacists, pharmacy technicians and pharmacy assistants. For example, it simplifies the understanding of dosage types (single, daily and total), extemporaneous preparations, alligation calculation, and dilution of concentrated formulations. In fact, it presents a unique and simplified way of understanding pharmaceutical calculations and computing. This book is highly recommended for educational institutions that offer healthcare courses involving pharmacy calculations.

Professor Faith-Michael Uzoka

CONTENTS

CHAPTER 1

Proportion: The Center of Mathematical Calculations in Pharmacy

Objectives

At the end of this chapter, students should be able to do the following:

- Demonstrate understanding of the concept of proportion
- Be in a position to outline the rules governing proportional calculations
- Apply the concepts of proportion in both pharmacy and everyday calculations

Introduction

Proportion is the relationship that exists between the size, number, quantity, value, amount, et cetera, of two or more variables. The concept of proportion is at the center of medical, pharmacy, and nursing math calculations. It seeks to establish the relationship between two or more values and thus extrapolate the same relationship to higher values or lower values than already provided. Most calculations in the medical profession can be successfully accomplished using the concept of proportions.

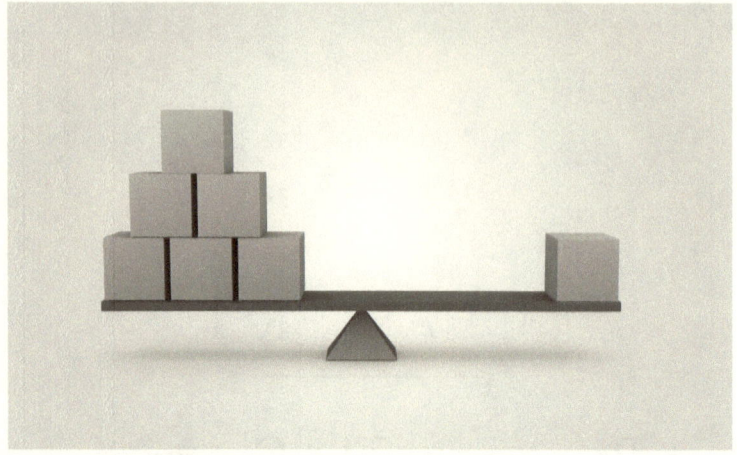

FIGURE 1.1 ***The Proportion:*** Proportion is all about the relationship that exists between the size, number, quantity, value or amount of 2 or more variables. The single box on the right has weight equivalence of the six boxes on the left.

1 box (R) →6 Boxes (L) OR 6 Boxes (L) → 1 Box (R)

Examples

If it is said that 1 teaspoon (tsp) is equivalent to 5 milliliters (mL), this is a proportional statement establishing the relationship between teaspoon and milliliter. In our proportional expressions, we can write this as:

$$1 \text{ tsp} \rightarrow 5 \text{ mL}$$

or

$$5 \text{ mL} \rightarrow 1 \text{ tsp}$$

If these statements are true, then

$$2 \text{ tsp} \rightarrow 10 \text{ mL } (5 \text{ mL} + 5 \text{ mL})$$
$$3 \text{ tsp} \rightarrow 15 \text{ mL } (5 \text{ mL} + 5 \text{ mL} + 5 \text{ mL})$$
$$0.5 \text{ tsp} \rightarrow 2.5 \text{ mL}$$

The expression "60 minutes make 1 hour" is a proportional statement establishing the relationship between minutes and hours. In our proportional expression, we can write this:

60 minutes → 1 hour

or

1 hour → 60 minutes

If these statements are true, then

120 minutes → 2 hours

240 minutes → 4 hours

30 minutes → 0.5 hours

...and so on.

If a pharmacy's telephone company charges the pharmacy $0.30 for every 2 minutes of outgoing calls, there you find a proportion establishing the relationship between the costs incurred by the pharmacy against a period of time. In our mathematical expression, we can write this as:

$0.30 → 2 minutes

or

2 minutes → $0.30

If these statements are true, then

$0.60 → 4 minutes

$1.20 → 8 minutes

$0.15 → 1 minute

...and so on.

If a pharmacist is traveling in his car at a constant speed of 50 kilometers (km) per hour (hr) [50 km/hr], a proportion is seen establishing the relationship between the distance the car covers (km) and the length of time it takes the car to cover it (hr).

Proportionally, we can say

50 km ➔ 1 hr

or

1 hr ➔ 50 km

If these are correct, then the following should also be true:

2 hrs ➔ 100 km

5 hrs ➔ 250 km

0.5 hr ➔ 25 km

. . . and so on.

With the proportions as established above, we can actually determine the distance the car travels over a given time or the time it will take the car to cover a certain given distance, as we shall see shortly.

A statement that a particular antibiotic suspension contains 3 milligrams (mg) of the medication (active ingredient) in every 5 mL of the suspension (3 mg / 5 mL) is one of proportion, establishing the relationship between the volume of the suspension (in milliliters) and the amount of active ingredient (in milligrams) it contains. Mathematically, we can represent the relationship as either

5 mL suspension ➔ 3 mg of medication

or

3 mg of medication ➔ 5 mL suspension

If these are true, then

10 mL suspension ➔ 6 mg of medication

20 mL suspension ➔ 12 mg of medication

2.5 mL suspension → 1.5 mg medication

... and so on.

This means that we can actually determine the amount of active medication (mg) when the volume of suspension is given. We can also calculate the volume of suspension (in milliliters) that will contain a given amount of active ingredient using the concept of proportion.

If a certain cream contains 8 grams (g) of the active medication in every 100 g of the formulation (8%), we can quickly see a sort of proportion established between the amount of active ingredient (in grams) and the amount of the entire cream formulation (also in grams) that contains it. Proportionally, we can say:

100 g formulation (cream) → 8 g active ingredient

or

8 g active ingredient → 100 g cream formulation

From the proportional statements above, it can be inferred that

200 g formulation → 16 g active ingredient

50 g formulation → 4 g active ingredient

25 g formulation → 2 g active ingredient

This means that we can indeed calculate the amount of active medication when the quantity of cream (formulation) is known, and we can also calculate the quantity of cream that can yield a given amount of active medications using the concept of proportions.

The list of such proportional relationships is apparently endless and is very common in medical calculations. Whenever two values are linked up in a relationship, a proportional knot will be patently established. Whether your paycheck is $700 every two weeks or you save $50 for your child's education every month or 1 gram of peanut costs 35 cents in a Superstore or 1 liter of gas costs $1.19 in Costco or every 5 mL of a liquid medicinal formulation provides 100 mg of the active ingredient.

These are all proportional statements. Most calculations involving medications and doses have something to do with proportion, and this will be seen throughout this book. Mastering proportional calculations is the key to excelling in such calculations.

At this point, students should be able to provide their own examples of such proportional statements.

The Calculations Proper

If seven days make one week

i.e.,

$$7 \text{ days} \rightarrow 1 \text{ week}$$

It is very easy to predict, through mental math, that

$$14 \text{ days} \rightarrow 2 \text{ weeks}$$
$$21 \text{ days} \rightarrow 3 \text{ weeks}$$
$$28 \text{ days} \rightarrow 4 \text{ weeks}$$
$$35 \text{ days} \rightarrow 5 \text{ weeks}$$

However, if pharmaceutical company makes a profit of 31.39 cents for every $8.02 revenue:

That is,

$$\$8.02 \text{ revenue} \rightarrow 31.39 \text{ cents profit,}$$

without applying any sort of formula, it will take an exceptional mathematical mind to predict the exact profit of this company if their total revenue is $699.93. Therefore, we need to establish a proportional formula that can lead us to the exact answer, no matter what type of fractions or decimals are involved.

$8.02 revenue → 31.39 cents profit

$699.93 revenue → unknown

The layout above is typical for most pharmacy calculations, where three values are provided (or implied) and the fourth (the unknown) will be required to be calculated.

Rules for Calculations Involving Proportions

Before we proceed to the calculations proper, we need to itemize the rules for solving proportional problems. In order to lay bare these rules, let us consider this question:

Example

If it is known that every 5 mL of a certain suspension (a kind of liquid formulation) contains 8 mg of the active ingredient, how many milliliters of the suspension will contain 40 mg of the active ingredient?

Solution

Rule 1. Establish the relationship between the two variables in the question.

First of all, we establish the relationship between the two variables (milliliters and milligrams) in the question. From the question, it is a fact that every 5 mL of the suspension contains 8 mg of the active ingredient. This is the relationship. Our first line of proportion will be

5 mL suspension → 8 mg medication

or

8 mg medication → 5 mL suspension

Note: These are called lines of proportion (the given). If A has a certain relationship with B, it means B also has the same relationship with A. Both statements mean the same. We will see shortly why one of the lines of proportion may be preferred over the other in solving a given calculation problem.

Rule 2. Always keep the unknown entity (what you are looking for) to the right.

Now there are two variables—milliliters (volume of suspension) and milligrams (amount of active ingredient). The question is asking for the *milliliters* (volume of suspension) that will contain 40 mg of active ingredient. So 40 mg is given, but the milliliter equivalent is unknown. The preferred line of proportion for solving this problem will be

$$8 \text{ mg medication} \rightarrow 5 \text{ mL suspension}$$
$$40 \text{ mg medication} \rightarrow \text{Unknown}$$

Rule 3. While solving for the unknown, make sure the units of the given (provided) variable are the same. If they are not the same, we must convert one to make both the same.

In the current example, the provided variables are 8 mg and 40 mg. They have the same unit; therefore the calculation can proceed.

From the current example,

$$8 \text{ mg medication} \rightarrow 5 \text{ mL suspension}$$
$$40 \text{ mg medication} \rightarrow u \text{ (unknown)}$$

But if, for example, 40 mg was given in its g equivalent (0.04 g), we must convert that value to milligrams to match with the other given unit. Please see chapter 2, "Interconversion of Units."

Rule 4. Solve your calculations.

Solving the current calculation goes like this:

$$8 \text{ mg medication} \rightarrow 5 \text{ mL suspension}$$
$$40 \text{ mg medication} \rightarrow u \text{ (u=unknown)}$$

$$u = \frac{5\ mL\ suspension}{8\ mg\ medication} \times \frac{40\ mg\ medication}{1}$$

=25 mL suspension

So as long as all the rules are observed and the calculations are spread out properly, it is always

$$\frac{Upper\ right}{Upper\ left} \times \frac{Bottom\ left}{1}$$

That is to say, if

$$A_1 \rightarrow B_1$$
$$A_2 \rightarrow u$$
$$u = \frac{B_1}{A_1} \times \frac{A_2}{1}$$

as long as A_1 and A_2 have the same unit and are referring to the same entity.

In one of our classes, one of my students was quick to ask for a proof of this formula. "Why not the other ways?" the student asked.

This is the proof.

Considering the example above, if

$$8\ mg\ ^{A1} \rightarrow 5\ mL\ ^{B1}$$

Then

$$16\ mg \rightarrow 10\ mL$$
$$24\ mg \rightarrow 15\ mL$$
$$32\ mg \rightarrow 20\ mL$$

$$40 \text{ mg}^{A2} \rightarrow unknown \text{ (= 25 mL)}$$

$$64 \text{ mg} \rightarrow 40 \text{ mL}$$

It is clear from above that at every line of proportion, values on the left divided by value on the right (or vice versa) will always give the same quotient, a constant.

$$\frac{8}{5} = \frac{16}{10} = \frac{24}{15} = \frac{32}{20} = \frac{\mathbf{40}}{\mathbf{u}} = \frac{64}{40} = 1.6 = \text{Constant}$$

This is as long as all numerators have the same unit, referring to the same entity, and all denominators have the same unit and are referring to the same entity. Therefore, to search for unknown (u) (i.e., the volume that corresponds with the 40 mg as the calculation demands), let us attach labels to the entities (see labels above).

$$\frac{8 \text{ mg (A1)}}{5 \text{ ml (B1)}} = \frac{40 \text{ mg (A2)}}{unknown}$$

Going with labels

$$\frac{A1}{B1} = \frac{A2}{u}$$

Cross-multiplying

$$A1 \times u = B1 \times A2$$

$$u = \frac{B1 \times A2}{A1}$$

$$= \frac{B1}{A1} \times \frac{A2}{1}$$

The value for u (from the formula above) corresponds with our earlier formula as long as A1 and A2 are the same entity with the same unit.

Substituting above will give us

$$\frac{5\ mL}{8\ mg} \times \frac{40\ mg}{1} = 25\ \text{mL}$$

Note: This formula only works if we place the unknown entity to the right of the proportional line. The units of the known (8 mg and 40 mg) must be the same and referring to the same entity. If these rules are observed, we are sure to arrive at the correct answer, and the unit of the answer would be the same as the unit of the top left numerator.

Now we can complete the profit calculation for the pharmacy that recorded total revenue of $699.96 and makes 31.39 cents profit for every $8.02 sales revenue.

$$\$8.02\ revenue \rightarrow 31.39\ \text{cents profit}$$

$$\$699.93\ revenue \rightarrow \text{unknown (u)}$$

(Watch the values to the left of the lines of proportion closely; they both have the same unit [$] and are both referring to the same entity [revenue].)

$$u = \frac{31.39\ cents\ profit}{\$8.02\ revenue} \times \frac{\$699.93\ revenue}{1}$$

$$= 2{,}739.50\ \text{cents}$$

Note: The answer must be in cents because the unit of the profit in our line of proportion is cents.

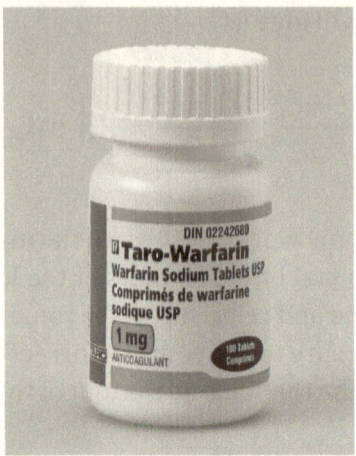

FIGURE 1.2 ***Taro-Warfarin 1 mg per Tablet:*** Each tablet contains 1 mg of the active ingredient warfarin. Each tablet weighs more than 1 mg because other non-active ingredients (bulking agents, disintegrants, lubricants, colorants, binders, etc.) are contained in each tablet. The 1 mg represents only the amount of the active ingredient in each tablet.

1 tab → 1 mg warfarin

(Courtesy Taro pharmaceuticals)

Example 1.1

Mrs. Anderson is a pharmacist who loves to bake for her family. Every 25 pancakes she makes require the use of 3 eggs. Help Mrs. Anderson calculate how many eggs are needed to make 100 pancakes.

Solution

Realize that this proportion is talking about the relationship between the number of eggs needed to make a certain number of pancakes. So the proportion can be represented mathematically as either

3 eggs → 25 pancakes

or

25 pancakes → 3 eggs

The question is asking about eggs (how many eggs?), so the unknown is the egg. Therefore, our line of proportion will present the eggs on the right-hand side.

If   25 pancakes → 3 eggs

Then   100 pancakes → u

$$u = \frac{3\ eggs}{25\ pancakes} \times \frac{100\ pancakes}{1}$$

$$= 12\ eggs$$

Note: When we write down our values ready for calculation, be sure to confirm that the unit of the numerator top right (in this case, pancake) should cancel out the unit of the lower-left denominator (pancake), leaving only the unit of the left numerator (eggs) as the unit for the emerging answer. If this does not happen, then certain rules of the proportional calculation might have been overlooked.

Example 1.2

Andy is an Ethiopian-born pharmacy assistant who practises in Calgary. Andy calls his friends regularly in Ethiopia, and the telephone company charges him 31.039 cents for every 0.8 minutes of phone call.

(a) What will be Andy's bill if he calls Ethiopia for one hour?
(b) If his budget in a month for telephone calls to Ethiopia is $25.00, how many minutes will that correspond to?

Solution

(a) Here we are looking for amount (bill), so the value corresponding to the money part will be on the right of our lines of proportion

0.8 minutes → 31.039 cents

This is establishing the relationship and, at the same time, placing the money part on the right side of the line of proportion (rule 1 and 2).

Now 1 hour indicates a time frame, but in a different unit than the minutes. Therefore, it must be converted to minutes to correspond to the unit in our established line of proportion (1 hour = 60 minutes) (rule 3).

So to continue,

$$0.8 \text{ minutes} \rightarrow 31.039 \text{ cents}$$

$$60 \text{ minutes} \rightarrow u$$

$$u = \frac{31.039 \text{ } cents}{0.8 \text{ } minutes} \times \frac{60 \text{ } minutes}{1}$$

$$= 2{,}327.925 \text{ cents}$$

This can be converted to dollars as $23.28

(b) The second part of the question is asking about the amount of time in minutes that $25.00 can fetch.

In this case, our line of proportion will have to be turned around to keep the minutes part at the right-hand side. Thus,

31.039 cents → 0.8 minutes (rule 1 and 2)

Now the $25.00, even though it indicates an amount, is in a different unit than the one in our established line of proportion. Hence the dollar must be converted to cents (rule 3).

$$\$25.00 = 2{,}500 \text{ cents}$$

Continuing

$$31.039 \ cents \rightarrow 0.8 \ minutes$$

$$2,500 \ cents \rightarrow u$$

$$u = \frac{0.8 \ minutes}{31.039 \ cents} \times \frac{2,500 \ cents}{1}$$

$$= 64.44 \ minutes$$

So with the monthly budget of $25.00, the expectation will be that Andy can make calls for only 64.44 minutes per month.

Example 1.3

An antihypertensive agent contains 5 mg of the active ingredient per tablet. How many tablets would be necessary to supply 55 mg of the active ingredient?

Solution

Here we are looking for the number of tablets, so tablets will be in the right of the line of proportion.

$$5 \ mg \rightarrow 1 \ tablet$$

$$55 \ mg \rightarrow u$$

$$u = \frac{1 \ tablet}{5 \ mg} \times \frac{55 \ mg}{1}$$

$$= 11 \ tablets$$

Note: Always attach units to your values. It will definitely guide us to ensure we are working with same units, and it will clearly indicate the unit of our final answer.

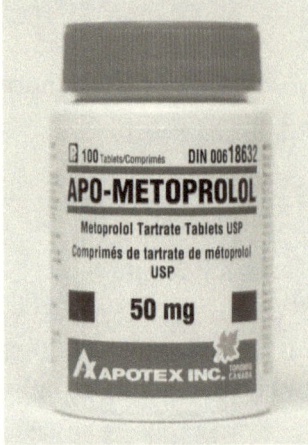

FIGURE 1.3 *Apo-Metoprolol Tablet 50 mg:* Each tablet of this medication contains 50 mg of the active ingredient metoprolol. There is thus a proportional relationship between the number of tablet and the amount of active ingredient contained.

1 tablet → 50 mg metoprolol OR 50 mg metoprolol → 1 tablet (Courtesy Apotex)

Example 1.4

An antiemetic suspension such as Gravol (dimenhydrinate) contains 125 mg of the medication in every 5 mL of the suspension. The physician wants 400 mg of the medication be given to the patient per dose. How many milliliters should that be?

Solution

We are obviously looking for milliliters in this case, so our lines of proportion should have mL on the right-hand side. Thus,

$$125 \text{ mg} \rightarrow 5 \text{ mL}$$

$$400 \text{ mg} \rightarrow u$$

$$u = \frac{5 \ mL}{125 \ mg} \times \frac{400 \ mg}{1}$$

$$= 16 \text{ mL}$$

So in order to administer 400 mg of the active ingredient to the patient, we must give 16 mL.

Note: The only unit left after cancellation is the mL, so the answer should be in milliliters.

Example 1.5

A certain compounded liquid medication for ulcer (omeprazole suspension) contains 8 mg of the medication in every 3 mL of the liquid. The pharmacy technician mistakenly spilled 18 mL on the floor while he was packaging the medication for the patient. How much of the medication (in milligrams) was lost because of that spill?

Solution

Again we are looking for the amount of medication in milligrams, so our line of proportion should have mg on the right.

$$3 \text{ mL} \rightarrow 8 \text{ mg}$$

$$18 \text{ mL} \rightarrow u$$

$$u = \frac{8 \ mg}{3 \ mL} \times \frac{18 \ mL}{1}$$

$$= 48 \text{ mg}$$

So 48 mg was lost by spilling 18 mL of the liquid.

Example 1.6

A certain compounded diclofenac gel (used for pain and inflammation) contains 7 grams of diclofenac powder in every 100 g of the gel. If 60 g of the gel were dispensed to a patient, what amount of diclofenac powder in grams will be contained in it?

Solution

We are looking for the amount of the active ingredient, so that should be on the right.

$$100 \text{ g gel} \rightarrow 7 \text{ g diclofenac}$$

$$60 \text{ g gel} \rightarrow u$$

$$u = \frac{7 \ g \ diclofenac}{100 \ g \ gel} \times \frac{60 \ g \ gel}{1}$$

$$= 4.2 \text{ g diclofenac powder}$$

Note: This is a special situation where both sides of a line of proportion have the same units (grams). However, to distinguish the different variables, we attach suffixes like *gel* and *diclofenac* so that each value can easily be identified.

Example 1.7

Novorapid insulin comes in the strength of 100 units/mL. The physician requires the patient to inject 35 units after each meal. How many milliliters should the patient inject after each meal?

Solution

We are looking for milliliters, so our line of proportion should have mL on the right.

$$100 \text{ units} \rightarrow 1 \text{ mL}$$

$$35 \text{ units} \rightarrow u$$

$$u = \frac{1 \ mL}{100 \ units} \times \frac{35 \ units}{1}$$

$$= 0.35 \text{ mL}$$

So the patient should inject 0.35 mL after each meal in order to receive 35 units of the Novorapid insulin.

Example 1.8

A certain cough syrup contains 100 mg of the active drug (dextromethorphan) in every 5 mL of the syrup. The physician's instruction says that the patient should take 150 mg of the active ingredient four times daily for 10 days.

a) How many milliliters should the patient take per dose (at one time)?
b) How many milliliters should the patient take per day?
c) How many milliliters should the patient take for the entire course of therapy?

Solution

Note: It is very important to focus on the question asked and dismiss nonrelevant and unnecessary information.

a) This question is asking for the amount (in milliliters) that the patient takes per dose (one-time consumption). Our line of proportion should have mL at the right-hand side.

$$100 \text{ mg active ingredient} \rightarrow 5 \text{ mL syrup}$$
$$150 \text{ mg active ingredient} \rightarrow u$$

$$u = \frac{5 \text{ mL syrup}}{100 \text{ mg active ingredient}} \times \frac{150 \text{ mg active ingredient}}{1}$$

$$= 7.5 \text{ mL per dose}$$

So patient takes 7.5 mL of the syrup (150 mg) per dose.

b) Patient therefore takes

$$7.5 \text{ mL} \times 4 = 30 \text{ mL per day}$$

c) Patient takes

$$30 \text{ mL} \times 10 = 300 \text{ mL for the entire course of therapy}$$

Example 1.9

A certain drug powder costs 49.6 cents per 3 kg of the powder. If a pharmaceutical company has mapped out a budget of $2,000 for the drug powder, what is the weight of powder they can buy?

Solution

Question is asking for weight of powder, so our weight is kept on the right-hand side.

$$49.6 \text{ cents} \rightarrow 3 \text{ kg}$$

The amount of $2,000 must be converted to cents to give it the same unit as is found in our line of proportion.

$$\$2,000 = 200,000 \text{ cents}$$

Continuing

$$49.6 \text{ cents} \rightarrow 3 \text{ kg}$$

$$200,000 \text{ cents} \rightarrow u$$

$$u = \frac{3 \ kg}{49.6 \ cents} \times \frac{200,000 \ cents}{1}$$

$$= 12,096.774 \text{ kg}$$

Example 1.10

A certain pharmacy makes a profit of 90.52 cents for every sale of $78.00.

a) How much profit in dollars will the pharmacy make if it recorded sales of $2,028.00 at the end of the day?
b) If the pharmacy's target is to make a profit of $35,000 at the end of the year, what will be their sales target for the year in dollars?

Solution

a) This question is asking about the profit, so we keep profit at the right side of our line of proportion.

$78.00 sales → 90.52 cents profit

$2,028 sales → u

$$u = \frac{90.52 \; cents \; profit}{\$78.00 \; sales} \times \frac{\$2,028 \; sales}{1}$$

=2,353.52 cents

Note: The answer is in cents because our line of proportion is in cents. This can be converted to dollars (as requested in the question) to $23.54.

b) This question is asking about sales, so we keep the sales in the right side of our line of proportion again.

90.52 cents profit → $78.00 sales

Now the given profit is in dollars, which represents amount but in a different unit than cents. Therefore we must convert the $35,000 to cents (Rule 3).

$35,000 = 3,500,000 cents

Continuing

90.52 cents profit → $78.00 sales

3,500,000 cents profit → u

$$u = \frac{\$78.00 \; sales}{90.52 \; cents \; profit} \times \frac{3,500,000 \; cents \; profit}{1}$$

=$3,015,908.08 sales

Note: The answer is in dollars because 'the sales' in the line of proportion is in dollars. Therefore, in order to make a profit of $35,000 in a year, the pharmacy must make a total sale of $3,015,908.08 in that year.

Chapter 1 Practice Questions

1. One ounce (oz) is considered to be equivalent to 30 mL. If a bowel has a capacity of 1,200 mL, how many ounces will fill the capacity?

2. If 50 tablets contain 1.5 g of active ingredient, how much of the ingredient in grams will be contained in 1,800 tablets?

3. Certain solution of an injectable medication comes as 100 mg of medication in every 2 mL. While preparing the injection for administration, the nurse wasted 0.8 mL. What amount of active ingredient in milligrams was wasted by the nurse?

4. A solution contains 50 mg of active ingredient in every 5 mL of the solution. How many milligrams will be contained in 1 tablespoonful? (1 tablespoonful=15 mL)

5. An antibiotic comes as a suspension of 250 mg / 5mL. If the patient needs 600 mg of the medication, how many milliliters should be administered?

6. A certain medication for arthritis comes as injectable suspension containing 0.5 mg / 2 mL. The dosage instruction says to give 4 to 8 mg intra-articular. What is the dosage range in milliliters?

7. Certain medication comes as tablets, each containing 0.5 mg of the active ingredient. The dosage instruction says to give a child 3 mg as crushed tablets. How many tablets must be crushed to deliver the 3 mg dose?

8. For every sale of $100 in a particular pharmacy, there is an expected profit of $11. What will be the expected profit when the pharmacy makes total sales of $1,500 in a day?

9. Dr. Hansen writes a prescription stating that he wants the patient to take 75 mg of the medication 3 times daily for 10 days. The stock bottle shows the medication contains 37.5 mg per tablet. How many tablets should the patient take in one day?

10. An antihypertensive medication contains 2.5 mg of the active ingredient per tablet. How many tablets would be necessary to supply a dose of 50 mg?

11. A cough syrup contains 60 mg of active ingredient in every 2.5 mL of syrup. The prescriber wants 100 mg be given to the patient. How many milliliters should be given?

12. The distance from the pharmacy to your house is 50 km. You normally travel at the speed of 25 km per hour. If you left your house by 8.00 a.m., what time are you expected to be at the pharmacy, all things being equal?

13. A patient spilled 50 mL of her medication. Her medication was labeled as 20 mg / 5 mL suspension. How many grams were lost as a result of the spill? (Note: 1,000 mg = 1 gram. See chapter 2)

14. If 24 pounds of a drug powder costs $48, what weight of the drug powder in pounds could be purchased with $78?

15. A certain medication has the dosage of 41 mg for every 3 m² body surface area of the child. If the child's total body surface is 42 m², what will be the child's dosage?

16. The cost of 120 tablets of aspirin is $0.96. How many tablets can $100.00 purchase?

17. If peanuts in Safeway stores go for 0.23 cents per pound. How much in dollars do you need in order to buy 24.8 pounds of the peanuts?

18. An elixir of acetaminophen contains 160 mg / 5 mL. How many milligrams would be used in preparing 1 ounce (30 mL) of the elixir?

19. A certain vaccine comes as injectable solution containing 1,000 units of the medication in every 3 mL of the solution. The dosage for the vaccine is 4 mL. How many units of the vaccine is one dose?

20. The standard indicates that 2.2 pounds is equivalent to 1 kg. What is the weight of a child in kilograms if the child's weight is 44 pounds?

21. A physician wrote a prescription for dexamethasone 20 mg/mL solution with the instruction to inject 0.75 mL intravenously. How many milligrams did the physician intend to be administered to the patient?

22. If a cough syrup contains 2 mg of codeine in each 5 mL dose, how much codeine in milligrams will be contained in 150 mL?

23. If a technician can travel in his car at a constant speed of 90 km per hour, how long will it take for the technician to reach Medicine Hat for a shift if he is coming from Calgary, which is a distance of 300 km?

24. A pharmacy decided to give back to customers as cashback $15 for every $100 a customer spent on a Tuesday, as a token for customer appreciation. If the total proceed on Tuesday is $940, how much will be the total amount given back as cashback to customers that day for appreciation?

25. Levemir insulin is available as an injectable containing 100 units of insulin/mL. If a physician requests a patient to inject 28 units, how many milliliters should that be?

26. If 150 gallons of a mouth rinse contain 30 grams of a coloring agent, how many grams of the coloring agent will be contained in 750 gallons?

27. Your energy company charges you $0.325 per 100 KJ of energy consumed. If you are given a bill of $16.25 at the end of the month, how many KJ of energy did you consume?

28. The dosage of a medication is 10 mg/kg body weight of a child. If the child weighs 28.6 kg, what will be the dosage in milligrams for the child?

29. If organic apples in Sobeys are sold at $0.23/pound, How many pounds of apples can you buy with $2.00?

30. How many milligrams of codeine would be in a tablespoonful of a medication containing a total of 50 mg codeine in a 60 mL bottle? (Hint: 1 tablespoonful = 15 mL)

31. A prescription instruction says to give 125 mg of the medication once daily. Available stock is in the strength of 250 mg per tablet. How many tablets should be given to the patient for 10 days of therapy?

32. If an entrepreneur pays his employees the total of $2,500 every two weeks, what will be the entrepreneur's budget for paychecks to employees in 2 years, assuming there are no pay increases and no change in number of employees? (Hint: 52 weeks make one year.)

33. If a pharmacist makes a savings of $28.56 every 2 weeks, how much will his total savings be in 3 years?

34. If the dosage of a drug for a man is 25 mg/kg, what will be the man's dose if he weighs 154 pounds? (Hint: 2.2 pounds = 1 kg)

35. If a physician instructs a nurse to inject 2 mL of dexamethasone labeled as 0.8 mg/mL, how much dexamethasone in milligrams was the physician intending to administer to the patient?

36. A physician prescribed amoxicillin 250 mg / 5 mL with the instruction to administer 200 mg. The nurse, however, administered 6 mL to the patient. What is the difference in milligrams between the physician's instruction and the actual amount administered to the patient?

37. A company projected that out of every $100 sales proceeds, $15 will go to charity as a donation. If the company wants to donate $480 to charity in a year, what will be their projected annual sales?

38. If one kilogram of a drug costs $0.98, what is the maximum kilogram of the drug that can be bought with $1,000.00?

39. A certain company discovered they lost $49.86 for every $100.00 they invested in that year. If their total loss was $99,720.00, how much was their total investment that year?

40. If one cup is equivalent to 240 mL, how many teaspoonfuls can fill a cup? (Hint: 1 tsp = 5 mL)

41. A physician wants the pharmacy to dispense 200 mg of amoxicillin per dose for a child. Amoxicillin is available as 125 mg / 5 mL suspension in the pharmacy. How many milliliters should be dispensed per dose?

42. If there are 9 foreign students for every 100 students in a certain pharmacy university, how many foreign students will there be if the total population of students in the said university is 900 students?

43. A patient's prescription states that the patient should receive 3 mg of active drug per kilogram of the patient's body weight. The patient weighs 50 kg. The drug is only available in 5 mg tablets. How many tablets should be administered to the patient?

44. If a pharmacist's constant speed is 80 km/hr along the Trans-Canada Highway, what distance would the pharmacist cover at that constant speed in 15 minutes?

45. One cup is considered equivalent to 240 mL. How many cups will fill up 1,200 mL?

46. If 15 gallons of a certain liquid costs $46.80, how much will 4 gallons cost?

47. If diarrhea remedy contains 3.9 mg of the drug in 35 mL of mixture, what amount of the drug in milligrams does 1 tsp (5 mL) of mixture contain?

48. A metered dose inhaler contains 250 mg of ipratropium bromide. If the inhaler can only deliver 200 sprays, how much of the drug in milligrams does each spray administer?

49. An elixir of sodium valproate (Epival) contains 40 mg of the active ingredient in every 5 mL of the liquid formulation. What amount of sodium valproate in milligrams will be contained in 400 mL of the elixir?

50. A physician orders 280 mg of cephalexin (Keflex) per dose for a child. The pediatric liquid medication contains 125 mg per 5 mL. How many milliliters should be given to the child for each dose?

A pharmacy technician has two bottles of different strengths of amoxicillin suspension.

Bottle A is 150 mL of amoxicillin suspension containing 250 mg of amoxicillin in every 5 mL.

Bottle B is 130 mL of amoxicillin suspension containing 125 mg of amoxicillin in every 5 mL.

He poured the contents of the two bottles in a bowl and mixed them thoroughly. Calculate the amount of amoxicillin that will be contained in every 5 mL of the resulting mixture.

Answers to Chapter 1
Practice Questions

1. 40 oz
2. 54 g
3. 40 mg
4. 150 mg
5. 12 mL
6. 16 to 32 mL
7. 12,500 tablets
8. $165
9. 6 tablets
10. 20 tablets
11. 4.167 ml
12. 10 AM
13. 0.2 g
14. 39 pounds
15. 574 mg
16. 12,500 tablets
17. $5.704
18. 960 mg
19. 1,333.333 units
20. 20 kg
21. 15 mg
22. 60 mg
23. 3.333 hours
24. $141
25. 0.28 mL
26. 150 g
27. 5,000 KJ
28. 286 mg
29. 8.696 lbs
30. 12.5 mg
31. 5 tablets
32. $130,000

33. $2,227.68
34. 1,750 mg
35. 1.6 mg
36. 100 mg
37. $3,200
38. 1,020.408 kg
39. $200,000
40. 48 teaspoon
41. 8 mL
42. 81 foreign students
43. 30 tablets
44. 20 km
45. 5 cups
46. $12.48
47. 0.557 mg
48. 1.25 mg
49. 3,200 mg
50. 11.2 mL

Solution to Star Question

When 130 mL suspension is mixed with 150 mL suspension, total volume becomes

$$130 \text{ mL} + 150 \text{ mL} = 280 \text{ mL}$$

So total resulting volume is 280 mL.

Next: What is the amount of medication (amoxicillin) in the entire mixture?

The amount of medication (amoxicillin) in the entire mixture is equal to amoxicillin from Bottle A + amoxicillin from Bottle B.

Amoxicillin from Bottle A (250 mg/5mL, 150 mL)

$$5 \text{ mL suspension} \rightarrow 250 \text{ mg amoxicillin}$$

$$150 \text{ mL suspension} \rightarrow u$$

$$u = \frac{250 \text{ mg amoxicillin}}{5 \text{ mL suspension}} \times \frac{150 \text{ mL suspension}}{1}$$

$$= 7,500 \text{ mg}$$

Amoxicillin from Bottle B (125 mg/5mL, 130 mL)

$$5 \text{ mL suspension} \rightarrow 125 \text{ mg amoxicillin}$$

$$130 \text{ mL suspension} \rightarrow u$$

$$= \frac{125 \text{ mg amoxicillin}}{5 \text{ mL suspension}} \times \frac{130 \text{ mL suspension}}{1}$$

$$= 3,250 \text{ mg}$$

So the total amoxicillin in milligrams contained in the mixture will be

$$7,500 \text{ mg} + 3,250 \text{ mg}$$

$$= 10,750 \text{ mg}$$

Therefore 10,750 mg of amoxicillin is contained in the mixture of 130 mL + 150 mL (= 280 mL). So we can draw our line of proportion

$$10,750 \text{ mg} \rightarrow 280 \text{ mL}$$

or

$$280 \text{ mL} \rightarrow 10,750 \text{ mg}$$

Now the question is, how many milligrams of amoxicillin will be contained in 5 mL of the resulting mixture? This means we are looking for milligrams inside 5 mL.

So we go:

$$280 \text{ mL suspension} \rightarrow 10{,}750\text{mg amoxicillin}$$

$$5 \text{ mL suspension} \rightarrow u$$

$$u = \frac{10{,}750 \; mg \; amoxicillin}{280 \; mL \; suspension} \times \frac{5 \; mL \; suspension}{1}$$

= 191.96 mg in every 5 mL of the new mixture

CHAPTER 2

Interconversion of Units

Objectives

At the end of this chapter, students should be able to do the following:

- Interpret the abbreviations for various units
- Identify international systems (SI) units or the metric system of measurement
- Recognize and identify the household units and systems of measurement
- Interconvert between the SI units and household systems of unit

Introduction

In whatever setting, a professional who works with medications should be able to identify the units attached to digits so as to know the precise values the digits are referring to. Measurements in the medical field rarely come without units. Measurement records without identifiable units are as confusing as a masked military personnel with weapons but no identifiable uniform in the war front.

The ability to place the correct units to our calculated answers is vital to pharmacy profession. For instance, a patient's dosage of 20 without a unit can be very confusing and has the potential of causing severe medication error. This is because the figure 20 may mean 20 tablets, 20 grams, 20 mL, or even 20 pounds. A correct figure without the correct unit is as well a source of potential danger.

All over the world, there are different systems used in the medical and pharmaceutical worlds to calculate drug amounts in weight and volume (and rarely length). In Canada, there are basically two systems used—the SI unit and the household system of units.

The *international system of units* (abbreviated SI), also known as the metric system, is derived from the French expression "Systeme International d'unites." These are the internationally accepted units of measurement based on *gram* (for weight), *meter* (for length), and *liter* (for volume).

The Canada Customary or household system of unit uses measurements such as teaspoon, tablespoon, and pint. This is commonly used in Canada, other North American countries, and even globally. Every health occupation professional who wishes to work with medication will do a lot of justice to him- or herself by being familiar with these measurements and how to identify and interconvert their values between other units of measurement.

The apothecary system has been used for many years in various disciplines when technology was less advanced. It employs units like grains, minims, drachms, et cetera, to express weight. It is used less frequently today due to inconsistency of values. In my several years of practice as a pharmacist in Canada, I have never seen a prescription with an apothecary unit of measure.

Measurement of Weight

Weight is the relative mass of a substance or the quantity of matter in it that gives rise to a downward force due to gravity. It can be described as the heaviness of a substance. The weight of a substance is determined by placing the material on a weighing scale or by comparing the weight of the sample material with standard weight(s) on a weighing balance. In pharmacy, weight is mainly used to express the amount of active ingredients in a formulation. It is also used to express the quantity of pharmaceutical susbtances, materials, solid and semi-solid formulations.

The SI Units of Weight

The international system of units for weight is based on the *gram*. The other units in the SI units are either multiples of the gram or its subdivision.

> 1,000 units (kilo)
>
> 100 units (hecto)
>
> 10 units (deka)
>
> *Gram*
>
> 0.1 units (deci)
>
> 0.01 units (centi)
>
> 0.001 units (milli)
>
> 0.000001 units (micro)

In Canada and other parts of North America, the most commonly used units are the gram, kilogram, milligram, and microgram. In SI unit, the gram is the basic measurement, and prefixes for the base measurement are used to indicate the multiples or submultiple of the base that is being described. So in this book, we will focus on the kilogram (kg), the gram (g), the milligram (mg), and the microgram (mcg).

$$\text{Milli} \rightarrow \text{one thousandth of a base } \left(\frac{1}{1,000}\right)$$

$$1\,g = 1,000\,mg$$

$$\text{Micro} \rightarrow \text{one millionth of a base } \left(\frac{1}{1,000,000}\right)$$

$$1\,g = 1,000,000\,mcg$$

$$\text{Kilo} \rightarrow \text{one thousand of a base } (1,000)$$

$$1\,kg = 1000\,g$$

The line of equivalency of the four common units for metric weight is shown below:

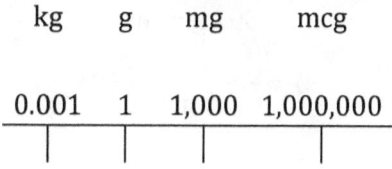

From above

$$0.001 \text{ kg} = 1 \text{ g} = 1,000 \text{ mg} = 1,000,000 \text{ mcg}$$

It is also clear that moving from kg →g →mg →mcg involves multiplying by 1,000 and moving from mcg →mg →g →kg involves dividing by a factor of 1,000. The following are worth memorizing by students:

1 kg → 1,000 g	OR	1,000 g → 1 kg
1 g → 1,000 mg	OR	1,000 mg → 1 g
1 mg → 1,000 mcg	OR	1,000 mcg → 1 mg

If these are memorized, any given unit in metric weight can be converted to another unit very easily by using the principle of proportion.

Example 2.1

Convert 500 g to its kilogram equivalent.

Solution

Here we employ the concept of proportion. The first question to ask ourselves is: what is the relationship between gram and kilogram? The answer will establish the relationship (rule 1)

We know that

$$1{,}000 \text{ g} \rightarrow 1 \text{ kg}$$

$$500 \text{ g} \rightarrow u$$

$$u = \frac{1 \, kg}{1{,}000 \, g} \times \frac{500 \, g}{1}$$

$$= 0.5 \text{ kg}$$

Note: We keep the kilogram to the right of the line of proportion (Rule 2) because we are looking for the kilogram equivalent of the given value in gram. Please see chapter 1 for rules of proportion calculation.

Example 2.2

Convert 5.4 kg to gram.

Solution

Here again, we first write down the relationship between gram and kilogram. We know that

$$1{,}000 \text{ g} \rightarrow 1 \text{ kg}$$

or

$$1 \text{ kg} \rightarrow 1{,}000 \text{ g}$$

In this case, we are looking for gram. The second line of proportion, which has gram on the right, becomes the one to use.

Hence,

$$1 \text{ kg} \rightarrow 1{,}000 \text{ g}$$

$$5.4 \text{ kg} \rightarrow u$$

$$u = \frac{1{,}000 \, g}{1 \, kg} \times \frac{5.4 \, kg}{1}$$

$$= 5{,}400 \text{ g}$$

Example 2.3

If a physician prescribed 30 g of an ointment, what is the milligrams equivalent of the weight prescribed?

Solution

Again, the first thing to do is to determine the relationship between gram and milligram.

We know that

$$1\text{ g} \rightarrow 1,000 \text{ mg}$$

(mg on the right because we want to convert to milligrams, having been given the quantity in grams)

$$30 \text{ g} \rightarrow \text{u}$$

$$\text{u} = \frac{1,000 \text{ mg}}{1 \text{ g}} \times \frac{30 \text{ g}}{1}$$

$$= 30,000 \text{ mg}$$

Example 2.4

Convert 0.3 mg to its gram equivalent

Solution

Likewise, first thing to do is to determine the relationship between milligram and gram, keeping the gram to the right (Rule 1 and 2 of proportion).

Thus,

$$1,000 \text{ mg} \rightarrow 1 \text{ g}$$

$$0.3 \text{ mg} \rightarrow \text{u}$$

$$u = \frac{1\,g}{1,000\,mg} \times \frac{0.3\,mg}{1}$$

$$= 0.0003 \text{ g}$$

Example 2.5

A particular strength of Synthroid comes as 100 mcg per tablet. What is the equivalence of 100 mcg in milligrams?

Solution

As usual, the first thing to do is to express the relationship between milligrams and micrograms in a line of proportion while keeping the milligrams on the right-hand side, thus,

$$1,000 \text{ mcg} \rightarrow 1 \text{ mg}$$

$$100 \text{ mcg} \rightarrow u$$

$$u = \frac{1\,mg}{1,000\,mcg} \times \frac{100\,mcg}{1}$$

$$= 0.1 \text{ mg}$$

Example 2.6

The order for a medication states that 0.01 mg of a drug powder should be administered to a patient immediately. If your scale can only measure in micrograms, how many micrograms should be administered to the patient?

Solution

Similarly, express the known proportional relationship between microgram and milligram first, while keeping the mcg at the right-hand side of the line of proportion.

Thus,

$$1 \text{ mg} \rightarrow 1{,}000 \text{ mcg}$$

$$0.01 \text{ mg} \rightarrow u$$

$$u = \frac{1{,}000 \; mcg}{1 \; mg} \times \frac{0.01 \; mg}{1}$$

$$= 10 \text{ mcg}$$

Example 2.7

A physician orders 0.002 kg of metformin to be given to a patient as a single dose. How many milligrams would the physician expect to be administered to the patient?

Solution

This can be solved in either of two ways:

Convert first to gram and then convert the answer to milligrams (two steps),

or

convert directly from kilogram to milligram (one step).

Option 1. Since

$$1 \text{ kg} \rightarrow 1{,}000 \text{ grams}$$

$$0.002 \text{ kg} \rightarrow u$$

$$u = \frac{1{,}000 \; grams}{1 \; kg} \times \frac{0.002 \; kg}{1}$$

$$= 2 \text{ g}$$

Then convert the 2 grams to milligrams.

$$1 \text{ g} \rightarrow 1{,}000 \text{ mg}$$
$$2 \text{ g} \rightarrow u$$
$$u = \frac{1{,}000 \text{ mg}}{1 \text{ g}} \times \frac{2 \text{ grams}}{1}$$
$$= 2{,}000 \text{ mg}$$

Therefore, 0.002 kg = 2,000 mg.

Option 2. We ask ourselves, what is the relationship between kilogram and milligram? Then we express that relationship as a line of proportion, with the milligrams on the right hand of the line of proportion.

$$0.001 \text{ kg} \rightarrow 1{,}000 \text{ mg}$$
$$0.002 \text{ kg} \rightarrow u$$
$$u = \frac{1{,}000 \text{ mg}}{0.001 \text{ kg}} \times \frac{0.002 \text{ kg}}{1}$$
$$= 2{,}000 \text{ mg}$$

Note that it may be easier to convert the units step-wise rather than making efforts to jump the ladder. It would be helpful for students to know the following lines of proportion by heart:

$$1 \text{ kg} \leftrightarrow 1{,}000 \text{ g}$$
$$1 \text{ g} \leftrightarrow 1{,}000 \text{ mg}$$
$$1 \text{ mg} \leftrightarrow 1{,}000 \text{ mcg}$$

As can be seen above, interconversion is possible among all the metric weight units. There is no metric weight unit that cannot be converted to another, either directly or step-wise. The reversal arrow means the equation can be reversed depending on what is being sought, keeping the unknown to the right.

Realize that

if

> 1 g → 1,000 mg
>
> 1,000 mg → 1 g

But

> 1,000 grams is not 1 mg

The SI Units of Volume

Volume is the capacity or the space occupied by a matter. In medical profession, liquid preparations are usually measured by volume. Some new students of nursing or pharmacy profession sometimes find it difficult to make the connection between volume and weight. In practice, the amount of active ingredients is usually expressed in weight (kilogram, gram, or milligram), and the space or amount of liquid where the ingredient is contained is usually expressed in volume (usually milliliter [mL]). For example, amoxicillin 250 mg / 5 mL means that every 5 mL (volume) of the suspension contains 250 mg (weight) of amoxicillin (the active ingredient).

The metric measurement (SI unit) of volume is based on liter (L). In practice, we commonly utilize the liter (L) and the milliliter (mL) in volume measurement. In this section, we will focus on these two units. The two units are related proportionally as shown below. When 1 liter is divided into 1,000 parts, 1 part of that is called 1 mL. The two are related proportionally, thus

> 1 L → 1,000 mL
>
> 1,000 mL → 1 L

The lines of proportion above are all that a student needs to memorize. With that known, you can convert from liters to millilters or milliliters to liters using the principle of proportion as discussed in chapter 1.

Example 2.8

Convert 0.3 L to its milliliter equivalent.

Solution

First is the relationship between liter and milliliter. Express this relationship as a line of proportion, leaving the mL on the right hand (because mL is unknown).

$$1 \text{ L} \rightarrow 1{,}000 \text{ mL}$$

$$0.3 \text{ L} \rightarrow u$$

$$u = \frac{1{,}000 \, mL}{1 \, L} \times \frac{0.3 \, L}{1}$$

$$= 300 \text{ mL}$$

Example 2.9

What is 70 mL expressed as liters?

Solution

Again, the question to ask is "What is the relationship between liter and milliliter?" Express that relationship as a line of proportion, keeping the liter to the right (because we are looking for the liter). Thus,

$$1{,}000 \text{ mL} \rightarrow 1 \text{ L}$$

$$70 \text{ mL} \rightarrow u$$

$$u = \frac{1 \, L}{1{,}000 \, mL} \times \frac{70 \, mL}{1}$$

$$= 0.07 \text{ L}$$

Example 2.10

A physician authorized 0.04 liters of a certain suspension to be dispensed to a patient. Your measuring cylinder is calibrated in milliliters. How many milliliters should you measure and dispense to the patient?

Solution

We are looking for the milliliter equivalent of a given liter.

$$1 \text{ L} \rightarrow 1,000 \text{ mL}$$

$$0.04 \text{ L} \rightarrow \text{u}$$

$$\text{u} = \frac{1,000 \text{ mL}}{1 \text{ L}} \times \frac{0.04 \text{ L}}{1}$$

$$= 40 \text{ mL}$$

In practice, to convert liters to milliliters, simply multiply by 1,000. To convert milliliters to liters, simply divide by 1,000. This is very important to know, as pharmacies and hospitals are fast-paced work places and working in such environments require appropriate time management skills.

Interconversion between Kilogram and Pound

The pound is one of the oldest units of weight. Up till now, we see patients' weight being expressed in pound in prescriptions where dosage calculations are based on the patient's weight in kilograms. It is therefore essential for the professional to be aware of how to interconvert between pound (lb) and kilogram (kg). This is because most dosages of medications are expressed per kilogram body weight while the patient's weight might be provided in pound. The relationship between pound and kilogram can be expressed as

$$2.2 \text{ pounds} \rightarrow 1 \text{ kg}$$

or

$$1 \text{ kg} \rightarrow 2.2 \text{ pounds}$$

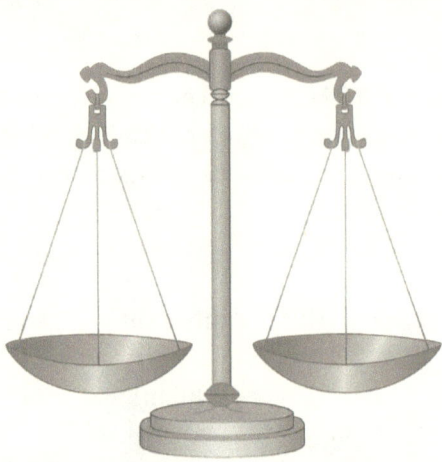

FIGURE 2.1 *The Weighing Balance:* The weighing balance is used to compare the weight of a specimen with a standardized known weight. Using this balance, approximately 2.2 pounds weight in one arm should balance a 1 Kg weight in the other arm.

With the lines of proportion above, any weight in the metric system can easily be converted to pound and vice versa.

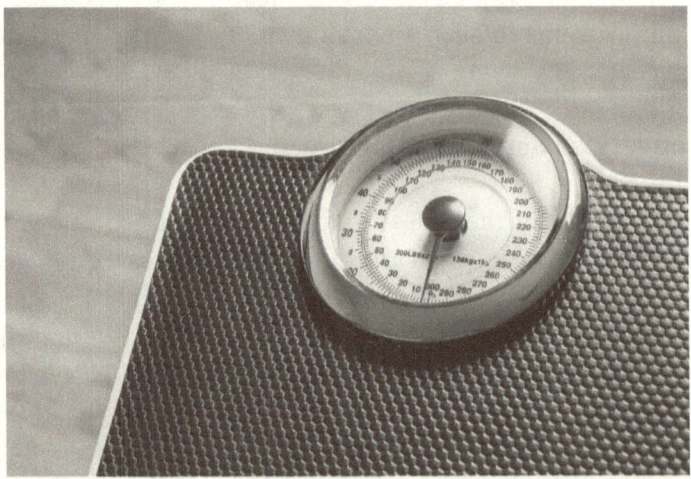

FIGURE 2.2 *The Clinical Weighing Scale:* The clinical weighing scale is used to measure the weight of humans or animals during clinical assessment. The calibration can be in kilogram, or pound or both (as in the picture above)

Example 2.11

If the weight of a child is 44 pounds, what is the child's equivalent weight in kilograms?

Solution

Now we are looking for the kilograms. Here we write our line of proportion such that kg will be on the right-hand side. Thus,

$$2.2 \text{ pounds} \rightarrow 1 \text{ kg}$$

$$44 \text{ pounds} \rightarrow u$$

$$u = \frac{1 \, kg}{2.2 \, pound} \times \frac{44 \, pound}{1}$$

$$= 20 \text{ kg}$$

Example 2.12

If a man's weight is 75 kg, what reading will the man expect on a weighing scale that is calibrated in pounds?

Solution

Again, we are looking for pounds, so our line of proportion will be drawn to reflect the pound on the right-hand side. Thus,

$$1 \text{ kg} \rightarrow 2.2 \text{ lbs}$$

$$75 \text{ kg} \rightarrow u$$

$$u = \frac{2.2 \, lbs}{1 \, kg} \times \frac{75 \, kg}{1}$$

$$= 165 \text{ lbs}$$

Example 2.13

If a physician ordered the dose of medication for a child to be 40 mg/kg body weight of the child and the child weighs 33 pounds, how many milligrams will the child's dose be?

Solution

As the dosage is presented in mg/kg and the child's weight in pounds, the first thing to do is convert the child's weight from pounds to kilograms to get the kilogram equivalent.

$$2.2 \text{ lbs} \rightarrow 1 \text{ kg}$$
$$33 \text{ lbs} \rightarrow u$$
$$u = \frac{1 \text{ kg}}{2.2 \text{ lbs}} \times \frac{33 \text{ lbs}}{1}$$
$$= 15 \text{ kg}$$

Therefore, the equivalent weight of the child is 15 kg.

Now the dosage calculation. For every kilogram body weight of the child, the child will receive 40 mg of the medication. This is a proportional relationship and can be represented thus:

$$1 \text{ kg} \rightarrow 40 \text{ mg}$$
$$15 \text{ kg} \rightarrow u$$
$$u = \frac{40 \text{ mg}}{1 \text{ kg}} \times \frac{15 \text{ kg}}{1}$$
$$= 600 \text{ mg}$$

Household or Canadian Customary System

The household unit of measure has, for a long time, remained a powerful tool for communication between health professionals. These measurements have long been taught and used in our daily life. The household measures are likely to be the measurements used in home settings for the administration of medications by patients. In the medical field, each household measure has been assigned a specific value in the metric system. This is in order to avoid errors of overdose or underdose.

For example, the teaspoon is one of the household measures but does not exactly mean the spoon we use to drink tea in our home (as the size of the teaspoon varies in different cultural settings). *In the medical field, a teaspoon only has the capacity of 5 mL.* If the doctor prescribes the dose of 1 teaspoon to the child, the only understanding is that the physician wants the patient to take 5 mL of the liquid medication, *just as 1 tablespoonful means 15 mL.* Another example of household measure is the cup. In the medical field, *one cup is considered to have a volume of approximately 240 mL* and has nothing to do with individual sizes of cups in our various homes. Most household measures are for volume measurement. Other household measures include drops, pints, gallons, and so forth.

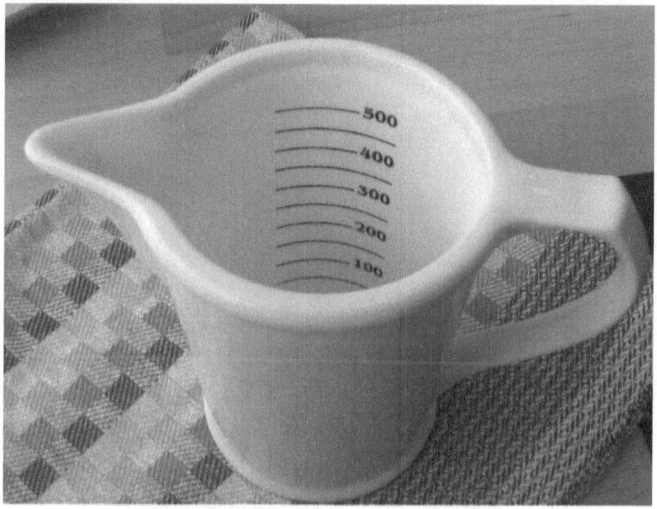

FIGURE 2.3 *The Calibrated Measuring Jug:* This is an example of a household measure for liquid formulations.

Some household measures and their metric equivalents

Measurement unit	Abbreviations	Metric equivalents	Equivalents
Teaspoon	tsp	5 mL	*100 drops
Tablespoon	tbsp	15 mL	3 tsp
Ounce	oz	30 mL	2 tbsp
Cup	c	240 mL	8 oz
Pint	pt	480 mL	2 cup
Quart	qt	960 mL	2 pt, 4 c
Gallon	Gal	3,840 mL	4 qt, 8 pt, 16 c
Drop	Gtts	*20 drops = 1 mL	*100 drops = 1 tsp

*   The size of a drop coming from a dropper is partly dependent on the size of the opening in the dropper and the viscosity of the dropping liquid. A wider dropper orifice leads to larger drop volume. The more viscous the liquid is, the larger the size of the drop, which means fewer drops can make large volume. In Canada and some parts of the world, for the purpose of certain dosage calculations involving drops, it is conventionally acceptable that 1 mL is equivalent to 20 drops from a standard dropper.

1 mL → 20 drops

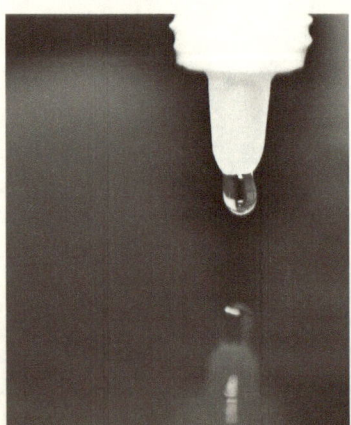

FIGURE 2.4 **The Drop:** The drop does not actually represent a specific volume and quantity of a liquid. The size of a drop coming out from a dropper orifice is partly dependent on the diameter of the dropper orifice and the viscosity of the dropping liquid. For calculation purposes, 1 mL is considered to yield 20 drops of the liquid from a standard dropper.

Example 2.14

A physician ordered amoxicillin 250 mg / 5 mL with the instruction to give 1 ½ teaspoon once daily to a child. How many milligrams does the physician want to be administered to the child daily?

Solution

We first need to convert the teaspoon value to milliliters because the strength of the suspension is expressed per milliliter.

$$1 \text{ teaspoon} \rightarrow 5 \text{ mL}$$

$$1.5 \text{ teaspoon} \rightarrow u$$

$$u = \frac{5 \ mL}{1 \ teaspoon} \times \frac{1.5 \ teaspoon}{1}$$

$$= 7.5 \text{ mL}$$

Then the next step is to find out how much amoxicillin in milligrams will be present in 7.5 mL of the suspension.

From the strength of the amoxicillin, it is clear that every 5 mL of the suspension contains 250 mg of amoxicillin. Keeping the milligrams part on the right-hand side, the proportional relationship will appear as follows:

$$5 \text{ mL} \rightarrow 250 \text{ mg amoxicillin}$$

$$7.5 \text{ mL} \rightarrow u$$

$$u = \frac{250 \ mg \ amoxicillin}{5 \ mL} \times \frac{7.5 \ mL}{1}$$

$$= 375 \text{ mg amoxicillin}$$

Therefore, in being given 1.5 teaspoons, the patient receives 375 mg of amoxicillin.

Example 2.15

A physician tells a patient who is scheduled for colonoscopy to drink 48 ounces of water 1 hour before his appointment. The patient does not have the measure for an ounce but has a standard measure for a cup. How many cups of water should the patient drink to follow the physician's order?

Solution

The question above is simply asking us to convert 48 ounces to cups.

$$48 \text{ ounces} = \underline{\hspace{2cm}} \text{ cups}$$

The best way to tackle this sort of question is to convert the ounces to its milliliter equivalent then convert that milliliter equivalent (which is technically 48 ounces) to cups.

Step one. Converting 48 ounces to milliliters.

We know that

$$30 \text{ mL} \rightarrow 1 \text{ ounce}$$
$$1 \text{ ounce} \rightarrow 30 \text{ mL}$$

Since we are looking for milliliters, the second line of proportion will be the preferred one to use.

$$1 \text{ ounce} \rightarrow 30 \text{ mL}$$
$$48 \text{ ounces} \rightarrow u$$

$$u = \frac{30 \text{ mL}}{1 \text{ ounce}} \times \frac{48 \text{ ounces}}{1}$$

$$= 1{,}440 \text{ mL}$$

Step two. Then convert the 1,440 mL to cups.

We know the relationship between milliliter and cup.

$$1 \text{ cup} \rightarrow 240 \text{ mL}$$

or

$$240 \text{ mL} \rightarrow 1 \text{ cup}$$

We use the second (preferred) as it has the cup on the right-hand side.

$$240 \text{ mL} \rightarrow 1 \text{ cup}$$

$$1,440 \text{ mL} \rightarrow u$$

$$u = \frac{1 \text{ cup}}{240 \text{ mL}} \times \frac{1,440 \text{ mL}}{1}$$

$$= 6 \text{ cups}$$

Therefore, 48 ounces = 6 cups

Example 2.16

A physician ordered 1.5 gallons of Colyte for a patient for stomach cleansing prior to a surgical procedure. The patient is not aware of the measurement called gallon. The patient wants to know the equivalence of 1.5 gallons in pints.

Solution

This question is simply asking us to convert 1.5 gallons to its pint equivalent.

$$1.5 \text{ gallon} = \underline{\hspace{1.5cm}} \text{ pint}$$

This can be comfortably solved in two steps.

Step 1. Convert the gallon to its equivalent volume in milliliter

Step 2. Convert the milliliter to its equivalent volume in pint

Step one.

$$1 \text{ gallon} \rightarrow 3{,}840 \text{ mL}$$

$$1.5 \text{ gallons} \rightarrow u$$

$$u = \frac{3{,}840 \, mL}{1 \, gallon} \times \frac{1.5 \, gallons}{1}$$

$$= 5{,}760 \text{ mL}$$

Step two. Convert the milliliters to pints.

$$480 \text{ mL} \rightarrow 1 \text{ pint}$$

$$5{,}760 \text{ mL} \rightarrow u$$

$$= \frac{1 \, pint}{480 \, mL} \times \frac{5{,}760 \, mL}{1}$$

$$= 12 \text{ pints}$$

Therefore, 1.5 gallon is equivalent to 12 pints.

The Apothecary System of Measurement

This is less often used in the contemporary setting, and its significance is gradually becoming historic. The apothecary system is one of the oldest systems of measurement, first used by the apothecaries (the pioneers of pharmacists). The apothecary units are gradually being completely replaced by the metric and household systems. The apothecary system uses units such as minims, fluid ounces, grains, drachms, and so forth. Exploration of the apothecary system is not within the scope of this book, and its relevance in contemporary pharmacy practice is gradually fading away. Students are encouraged to search relevant reference sources if they wish to know more about this historical system of measurement.

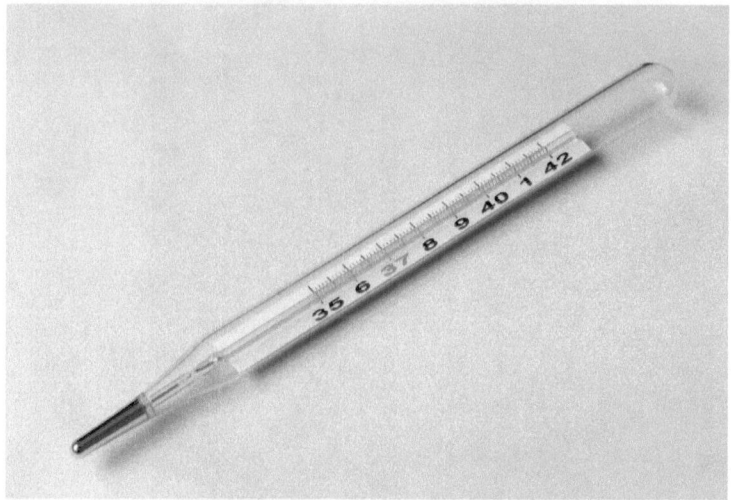

FIGURE 2.5 *The Clinical Thermometer:* The clinical thermometer uses thermometric liquids like alcohol or mercury to measure the body temperature of humans or animals. Temperature measurement can be oral, anal, or by placing the thermometer bulb in the underarm.

Interconversion of Temperature

Fahrenheit is a temperature scale that bases the boiling point of water at 212° and the freezing point at 32°. It was developed by Daniel Gabriel Fahrenheit, a German-born scientist. He discovered that, according to the scale he had marked on a thermometer, ice melted at 32° and water boiled at 212°, giving a difference of 180° between the freezing point and boiling point of water.

Sometime later, Anders Celsius, a Swedish astronomer, suggested the convenience of having a thermometer with a scale calibrated such that there will be a difference of 100° between two fixed points, with 0° for the freezing point of water and 100° for the boiling point of water. These two scales are still in use up till today.

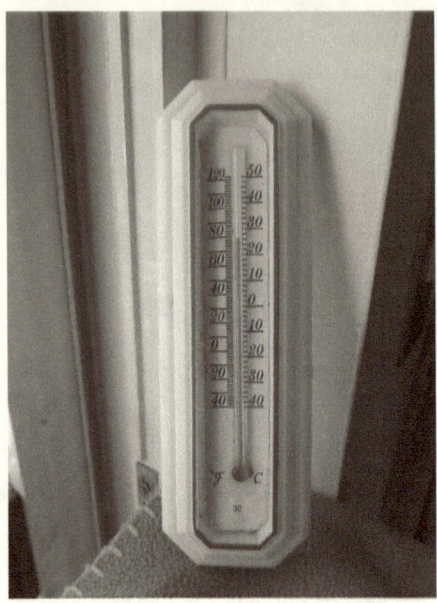

FIGURE 2.6 *The Dual Scale Thermometer:* Some thermometers are
calibrated in both Fahrenheit and Celsius for easy convertibility.

In Celsius (centigrade), there are 100° centigrade measuring the same
range of temperatures as 180° Fahrenheit. Each degree centigrade is
therefore equivalent to 1.8 or $\frac{9}{5}$ the size of each degree Fahrenheit.

From among the different arithmetic methods of converting
temperatures from Centigrade to Fahrenheit and vice versa, the
following formulas have been simplified

$$°F = \frac{9}{5}(°C) + 32$$

$$°C = (°F - 32) \times \frac{5}{9}$$

The knowledge of this conversion is important because some
thermometers in the pharmacy or hospital can be calibrated in either
of the scales.

Example 2.17

Convert 30°C to its corresponding degree in Fahrenheit.

Solution

$$°F = \frac{9}{5}(× 30) + 32$$

$$= 86°F$$

Example 2.18

Convert 86°F to its corresponding degree in centigrade

Solution

$$°C = (°F - 32) × \frac{5}{9}$$

$$= (86 - 32) × \frac{5}{9}$$

$$= 54 × \frac{5}{9}$$

$$= 30°C$$

Chapter 2 Practice Questions

1. Convert 100°F to its corresponding value in °C.

2. How many teaspoons are in 3 cups of liquid medication?

3. A physician's prescription is as follows: Amoxicillin 250 mg / 5 mL. Take 0.2 g 3 times daily. How many milliliters will supply the 0.2 g amoxicillin?

4. If the dosage of a drug is 50 mg/pound of patient's weight and the patient's weight is 55 kg, how many grams should be administered to the patient?

5. A physician writes a prescription for 2 pints of Benadryl. How many ounces should that be?

6. How many cups will fill up one quart?

7. A physician prescribes 0.75 kg of an ointment. How many grams does that represent?

8. If a physician orders Cefprozil 40 mg / kg body weight per day for a child and the child weighs 44 pounds, how many milligrams will be administered to the child?

9. In question 8 above, if the Cefprozil is labeled as 125 mg / 5 mL, how many milliliters should be given to the child per day?

10. Convert 100°C to its corresponding Fahrenheit temperature value.

11. How many teaspoons can fill up 3.5 ounces?

12. A patient bought 12 oz of liquid medication. He is scheduled to take 1 teaspoon every day. How long will the liquid medication last?

13. A medication is formulated as a patch, with each patch containing 25 micrograms. How many milligrams of the medication is contained in 5 patches?

14. A man told you his weight is 82 kg. You want to confirm this weight in your pharmacy with a scale that is calibrated in pounds. What weight in pounds will you be expecting?

15. Convert 0°F to its corresponding degree in centigrade.

16. The usual dose of a medication is 150 mg / kg body weight. How many milligrams should be administered to a patient weighing 154 pounds?

17. You are to dispense 300 mL of a liquid preparation. If the dose is 2 teaspoons, how many doses will the whole preparation contain?

18. A particular suspension is said to contain 125.8 mg of medication in every 10 mL of the suspension. How many grams are present in 5 mL of the suspension?

19. If a child's weight is 58 pounds, what is the equivalent weight in kilograms?

20. Convert 35°C to its corresponding degree in Fahrenheit.

21. If a patient takes 1 cup of medication 3 times a day, how many milliliters will the patient take per week?

22. Convert 98 pounds to its gram equivalent.

23. A tablet of Synthroid is marked 50 mcg. How many milligrams does that represent?

24. If a solution is labeled 7 mg / 5 mL, how many grams of the medication will be contained in 1 L of the solution?

25. Convert 108.7°F to its corresponding degree in centigrade.

26. If a patient's suspension is labeled 200 mg / 2 mL. The instruction is to take 1 teaspoon daily. How many milligrams are expected to be taken daily?

27. A patient has to be infused with 2 pints of blood. How many cups are equivalent to that volume?

28. A physician ordered 1.5 g of metformin to be administered to the patient. How many milligrams would the physician expect to be administered to the patient?

29. If a suspension is labeled 5 mg / 3 mL, how many micrograms are contained in 1.8 mL?

30. If a dose of a drug is 200 mg, how many doses are contained in 10 g?

31. A suspension is labeled 100 mg / 5 mL. How many grams of the active ingredient will be contained in 100 mL of the suspension?

32. Convert 4.4 pounds to its milligram equivalent

33. The thermometer used in measuring a child's temperature was calibrated in °C. The temperature reading was 39.5°C. What is the value of this temperature in °F?

34. A physician instructed that an antibiotic should only be administered if a child's temperature is constantly above 104.0°F. What is the Celsius conversion?

35. A physician authorized 4 liters of Colyte to a patient for colonoscopy. How many milliliters should be dispensed if the pharmacy stockkeeper's unit is in milliliters?

36. If an anti-infective liquid medication is labeled as 5 mg / 3 mL, how many milligrams will be contained in every tablespoonful?

37. A suspension contains 5 mg of medication per 3 mL of the suspension. How many milligrams are contained in 1 cup?

38. A bag of fluid must be given a body temperature of 37°C. What is the Fahrenheit conversion?

39. Convert 234 mL to its liter equivalent.

40. A child was supposed to take half a tablespoon of Zantac suspension. If the parents only have a teaspoon to measure, how many teaspoons should the parent administer to the child in order to deliver the accurate dose??

41. A tablet of Epival contains 500 mg of divalproex sodium. How would this be written in grams?

42. If a body fluid is to be stored at a temperature cooler than 60°F, what is the temperature for the storage in a refrigerator whose temperature is displayed on a Celsius thermometer?

43. A bag of powdered drug is marked as 925 g. How much is this weight if your scale in the pharmacy is calibrated in kilograms?

44. There is an order for 0.625 mg Premarin tablets. How many micrograms of medication will be contained in each tablet?

45. How many tablespoons will fill 1 pint?

46. How many milliliters will make up 0.5 L?

47. A physician instructs that a child should only take Tylenol if her temperature is higher than 39°C. What is the Fahrenheit conversion?

48. Express 0.234 grams in its microgram equivalent.

49. Clindamycin is available as 300 mg/capsule. How many grams of clindamycin does a capsule contain?

50. The dosage instruction of a liquid medication is 1 tablespoon three times daily for 10 days. How many ounces should be dispensed to the patient for the entire duration of the therapy?

★ Star Question ★

180.4 pounds = _____ mg?

Answers to Chapter 2
Practice Questions

1. 37.78°C
2. 144 teaspoons
3. 4 mL
4. 6.05 grams
5. 32 ounces
6. 4 cups
7. 750 grams
8. 800 mg
9. 32 mL
10. 212°F
11. 21 teaspoons
12. 72 days
13. 0.125 mg
14. 180.4 pounds
15. –17.778°C
16. 10,500 mg
17. 30 doses
18. 0.0629 gram
19. 26.36 kg
20. 95°F
21. 5,040 mL
22. 44,545.45 g
23. 0.05 mg
24. 1.4 g
25. 42.61°C
26. 500 mg
27. 4 cups
28. 1,500 mg
29. 3,000 mcg
30. 50 doses
31. 2 gram
32. 2,000,000 mg

33. 103.1°F
34. 40°C
35. 4,000 mL
36. 25 mg
37. 400 mg
38. 98.6°F
39. 0.234 L
40. 1.5 teaspoons
41. 0.5 gram
42. < 15.56°C
43. 0.925 kg
44. 625 mcg
45. 32 tablespoons
46. 500 mL
47. 102.2°F
48. 234,000 mcg
49. 0.3 gram
50. 15 ounces

Solution to Star Question

We convert the 180.4 pounds first to kilograms, then convert the kilograms to grams and then to its milligram equivalent.

$$2.2 \text{ pounds} \rightarrow 1 \text{ kg}$$

$$180.4 \text{ pounds} \rightarrow u$$

$$u = \frac{1\,kg}{2.2\,pounds} \times \frac{180.4\,pounds}{1}$$

$$= 82 \text{ kg}$$

Then convert the 82 kg to its gram equivalent.

$$1 \text{ kg} \rightarrow 1,000 \text{ grams}$$

$$82 \text{ kg} \rightarrow u$$

$$u = \frac{1,000 \text{ grams}}{1 \text{ kg}} \times \frac{82 \text{ kg}}{1}$$

$$= 82,000 \text{ grams}$$

Then convert the 82,000 grams to its milligram equivalent

$$1 \text{ gram} \rightarrow 1,000 \text{ mg}$$

$$82,000 \text{ grams} \rightarrow u$$

$$u = \frac{1,000 \text{ mg}}{1 \text{ gram}} \times \frac{82,000 \text{ grams}}{1}$$

$$= 82,000,000 \text{ mg.}$$

Therefore, 180.4 pounds = 82,000,000 mg

CHAPTER 3

Ratios and Percentages: Their Applications in Pharmaceutical Calculations

Objectives

At the end of this chapter, students should be able to do the following:

- Interpret ratio as expressed
- Demonstrate the understanding of percentages
- Apply the knowledge of ratio in solving simple pharmacy calculations
- Utilize the concept of percentages in solving simple pharmacy calculations
- Apply ratio and percentage principles in the continuum of proportional calculations

Introduction to Ratio

A ratio is a relationship between two or more parts of a whole or between one or more parts and a whole. In the course of the work of a pharmacist or allied professional, the knowledge and understanding of ratio will ultimately be needed in various calculations. When a pharmacy professional compounds certain products, they may be required to solve problems involving ratio. Proper understanding of ratio is therefore very essential to a pharmacist or pharmacy technician.

Understanding the ratio

If two different creams (cream A and Cream B) are blended together in a ratio of 2:3, the understanding is as follows:

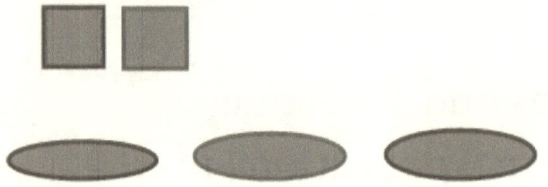

The square represents cream A, and the oval represents cream B.

The ratio can be represented as either

2:3   or   2 is to 3   or   2/3

What the ratio actually means is that for every 5 parts of the cream mixture, there are 2 parts of cream A and 3 parts of cream B. Realize that expressions of the ratio 2:3 as 2/3 can sometimes be confusing. The expression 2/3 does not mean the traditional two-third (2 out of every 3 shapes) but means 2 parts of A for every 3 parts of B or 2 parts of A out of every total of 5 parts of mixture, not 2/3 of the total number of parts. Because the two creams are measurable by weight, we can conveniently say that for every 5 gram of the mixture blend, there are 2 grams of cream A and there are 3 grams of the cream B.

Hence the ratio means that for every 5 grams of mixture, 2 grams are cream A and 3 grams are cream B.

5 gram mixture → 2 grams A and 3 grams B
10 gram mixture → 4 grams A and 6 grams B

20 gram mixture → 8 grams A and 12 grams B

And so on . . .

Realize too that the expression above has a form similar to the proportion we have already dealt with in early chapters. Using the expressions above, it will be easy to calculate the quantity of cream A if we know the total quantity of the entire cream mixture in question. It is also easy to predict the total quantity of the cream mixture if we have an idea of the quantity of cream A or cream B contained in the mixture.

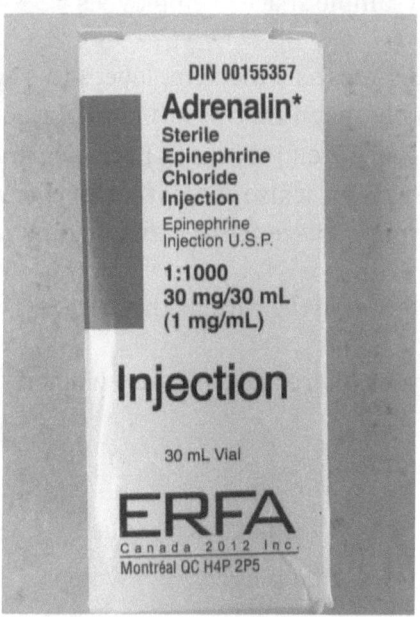

FIGURE 3.1 *The Ratio and Concentration Expression:* The expressed ratio of 1:1000 (one is to one thousand) is used to compare the proportion of the active ingredient to the quantity of formulation that contains the active ingredient. The "1" in the ratio expression (1:1000) represents one unit of the active ingredient while the "1000" represents 1000 units of the formulation. This means that 1000 mL of the formulation (solution) will contain 1 gram of the active ingredient – see chapter 4 (Courtesy ERFA)

Example 3.1

In a certain pharmacy, the ratio of men employees to women employees is 3:4. If the total number of employees is 210, how many employees are men, and how many employees are women?

Solution

Male employees	3
Women employees	4

(Total sample space of employees = 3 + 4 = 7)

Realize the ratio 3:4 means 3 men employees to 4 women employees but does not actually mean that ¾ are men. Rather, it means that 3 employees out of every 7 employees ($\frac{3}{7}$) are men and 4 out of every 7 employees ($\frac{4}{7}$) are women. It also means that for every 3 men employees you see in the pharmacy, there are 4 corresponding women employees.

The real interpretation of the ratio is this:

For 7 total employees, there are 3 men + 4 women

Or simply

7 employees → 3 men

7 employees → 4 women

Now depending on what is provided, we can actually calculate the number of men employees or women employees when we are provided with the total number of employees at the pharmacy. We can also calculate the expected total number of employees if we know the number of either men employees or number of women employees using proportion principles.

For the number of men employees,

7 total employees → 3 men employees

210 total employees → u

$$u = \frac{3\ men\ employees}{7\ total\ employees} \times \frac{210\ total\ employees}{1}$$

= 90 men employees

For the number of women employees,

7 total employees → 4 women employees

210 total employees → u

$$u = \frac{4\ women\ employees}{7\ total\ employees} \times \frac{210\ total\ employees}{1}$$

= 120 women employees

So for the 210 employees in the pharmacy, if the ratio of men to women is 3:4, there are 90 men employees and 120 women employees.

90 + 120 = 210

Example 3.2

In a certain university of pharmacy, the ratio of foreign students to indigenous students is 3:5. If the population of foreign student is 600:

(a) What is the expected total population of the school?
(b) What is the expected population of indigenous students?

Solution

Foreign   ●●●

] Total sample space is 8 students.

Indigenous   ○○○○○

What this ratio means is that for every 8 students, 3 are foreign and 5 are indigenous.

Proportionally, this can be represented thus:

8 total student population → 3 foreign
students + 5 indigenous students

That is,

8 total population → 3 foreign students

3 foreign students → 8 total population

or

8 total population → 5 indigenous students

5 indigenous students → 8 total population

Our calculation can be successfully accomplished using any of the lines of proportion above, provided we keep what we are looking for to the right-hand side of our chosen line of proportion.

First part of the question is asking for the total population of students, with the population of foreign students provided.

Hence the second line of proportion will be useful. (See chapter 1: proportion.)

Therefore,

3 foreign students → 8 student population

600 foreign students → u

$$u = \frac{8 \ student \ population}{3 \ foreign \ students} \times \frac{600 \ foreign \ students}{1}$$

= 1,600 total student population

To solve the second part of the question, we can subtract to get the population of indigenous students, like this:

Total student population = foreign students + indigenous students

1,600 = 600 + indigenous students

Indigenous students = 1,000

Or, we can also refer back to our line of proportion that will have the indigenous students at the right.

$$8 \text{ student population} \rightarrow 5 \text{ indigenous}$$

$$1{,}600 \text{ student population} \rightarrow u$$

$$u = \frac{5 \text{ indigenous}}{8 \text{ student population}} \times \frac{1{,}600 \text{ student population}}{1}$$

$$= 1{,}000 \text{ indigenous students}$$

Example 3.3

In a certain community where Jophil Pharmacy is located, the ratio of unemployed: employed: business people is 2:3:7.

If each person in the community can only belong to one of the groups at a time and the total population of this community is 4,800 people, what is the expected population of the unemployed, employed, and business people?

Solution

We can represent unemployed as U, employed as E, and business people as B.

$$U = \square\square$$
$$E = \square\square\square$$
$$B = \square\square\square\square\square\square\square$$

Total sample space is 12 people.

The expression means this: For every 12 individuals in the community, there are 2 unemployed, 3 employed, and 7 business persons.

That is,

Population 12 → 2 unemployed, 3 employed, 7 business people

Proportionally,

12 inhabitants → 2U

12 inhabitants → 3E

12 inhabitants → 7B

To calculate for U

12 inhabitants → 2 unemployed

4,800 inhabitants → u

$$u = \frac{2\ unemployed}{12\ inhabitants} \times \frac{4{,}800\ inhabitants}{1}$$

= 800 unemployed

To calculate for E

12 inhabitants → 3 employed

4,800 inhabitants → u

$$u = \frac{3\ employed}{12\ inhabitants} \times \frac{4{,}800\ inhabitants}{1}$$

= 1,200 employed

To calculate for B

12 inhabitants → 7 business people

4,800 inhabitants → u

$$u = \frac{7\ businesspeople}{12\ inhabitants} \times \frac{4{,}800\ inhabitants}{1}$$

= 2,800 business people

Therefore,

800 U + 1,200 E + 2,800 B = 4,800 total population of inhabitants

Example 3.4

A physician ordered a pharmacy to mix nystatin cream and Glaxal base at the ratio of 2:5 combinations. If the physician wants the pharmacist to supply only 140 grams of the mixture to the patient, how many grams of the nystatin cream and Glaxal base does the pharmacist need to mix?

Solution

$$
\left.
\begin{array}{l}
\text{Nystatin} \quad \bullet\bullet \\[12pt]
\text{Glaxal base} \quad \circ\circ\circ\circ\circ
\end{array}
\right] \text{Total 7 g}
$$

7 grams of mixture → 2 grams nystatin + 5 grams Glaxal base

7 g of mixture will need → 2 g nystatin

7 g of mixture will need → 5 g Glaxal base

Calculating for nystatin cream

7 g mixture → 2 g nystatin

140 g mixture → u

$$u = \frac{2\ grams\ nystatin}{7\ grams\ mixture} \times \frac{140\ grams\ mixture}{1}$$

= 40 grams nystatin cream

Calculating for Glaxal base

7 g mixture → 5 g Glaxal base

140 g mixture → u

$$u = \frac{5\ g\ Glaxal\ base}{7\ g\ mixture} \times \frac{140\ g\ mixture}{1}$$

= 100 g Glaxal base

40 g nystatin + 100 g Glaxal base

= 140 g mixture as ordered

Note: It is wise to attach labels identifying the components in the line of proportion so that it is easy to track which is which. This is because, as it can be seen, all the components have the same unit, gram, so labeling them as Glaxal base, nystatin or mixture assists in tracking them.

Example 3.5

A pharmacist mixed ethanol and distilled water at the ratio of 4 mL ethanol : 5 mL of distilled water homogeneously. How many milliliters of ethanol and how many milliliter of distilled water do you expect to find in 36 mL of the resulting mixture?

Solution

Ethanol ●●●● 4 mL

Distilled water ○○○○○ 5 mL

Total 9 mL

Every 9 mL of mixture contains 4 mL of Ethanol.

Every 9 mL of mixture contains 5 mL of distilled water.

9 mL mixture → 4 mL ethanol

9 mL mixture → 5 mL distilled water

Calculating for ethanol in 36 mL mixture

9 mL mixture → 4 mL ethanol

36 mL mixture → u

$$u = \frac{4\,mL\,ethanol}{9\,mL\,mixture} \times \frac{36\,mL\,mixture}{1}$$

= 16 mL ethanol

Calculating for distilled water

9 mL mixture → 5 mL distilled water

36 mL mixture → u

$$u = \frac{5 \; ml \; distilled \; water}{9 \; ml \; mixture} \times \frac{36 \; ml \; mixture}{1}$$

$$= 20 \text{ mL distilled water}$$

16 mL ethanol + 20 mL Distilled water = 36 mL mixture

Example 3.6

A pharmacist set out to prepare a 200 g mixture of Hyderm cream and Fucidin cream in a combination ratio of 2:3. Before the pharmacist started making the compound, he found out that he has only 30 g of Fucidin and enough nystatin to satisfy the ratio. What is the maximum amount of the mixture he can make with the available 30 g Fucidin cream, and what amount of nystatin cream will be used in making the mixture?

Solution

Fucidin cream   ●● 2 g

Hyderm cream   ооо 3 g

Total 5 g

From the demonstration above, it is clear that every 5 g of the mixture will contain 2 g Fucidin cream, and every 5 g of the mixture will contain 3 g of Hyderm cream. And for every 2 g of Fucidin, there must be 3 g of Hyderm cream to satisfy the ratio. These are statements of proportion and can be represented mathematically.

5 g mixture → 2 g Fucidin

5 g mixture → 3 g Hyderm

3 g Hyderm → 2 g Fucidin

We can use these lines of proportion to get what we are looking for. This time, we are looking for total mixture given the limited amount of Fucidin available.

So we can say

2 g Fucidin cream → 5 grams mixture (keeping the mixture component to the right because we are looking for mixture quantity in 30 g Fucidin)

30 g Fucidin cream → u

$$u = \frac{5\ g\ mixture}{2\ g\ fucidin} \times \frac{30\ g\ Fucidin}{1}$$

= 75 g mixture

So the pharmacist can only make a max of 75 g mixture using the available 30 g Fucidin.

Calculating for the amount of Hyderm needed to make the 75 g

5 g mixture → 3 g Hyderm

75 g mixture → u

$$u = \frac{3\ g\ Hyderm}{5\ g\ mixture} \times \frac{75\ g\ mixture}{1}$$

=45 g of Hyderm

So the pharmacist mixed the available 30 g Fucidin and 45 g Hyderm to make 75 g of the mixture at 2:3 ratio (Fucidine: Hyderm).

Example 3.7

A pharmacy technician mixed 160 mL of Ora-Blend syrup and 480 mL of simple syrup to make 640 mL of her own special oral vehicle for oral suspensions.

What is the ratio of Ora-Blend to simple syrup in her special mixture?

How many milliliters of Ora-Blend and simple syrup will be contained in every 5 mL of the mixture?

Solution

Part A

Ora-Blend syrup → 160 mL

Simple syrup → 480 mL

Ratio of Ora-Blend : Simple syrup

160 mL : 480 mL

This can further be reduced to its simplest form by dividing with common factors to get

1:3

So the ratio of Ora-Blend to simple syrup is

(1:3)

Ora-Blend   ● 1 mL ⎤
                            ⎥ Total 4 mL
Simple syrup   ooo 3 mL ⎦

Part B

From the expression above

Every 4 mL of the mixture contains 1 mL Ora-Blend.

Every 4 mL of the mixture contains 3 mL simple syrup.

4 mL mixture → 1 mL Ora-Blend

4 mL mixture → 3 mL simple syrup

Calculating for milliliters of Ora-Blend in 5 mL mixture

4 mL mixture → 1 mL Ora-Blend

5 mL mixture → u

$$u = \frac{1\ ml\ Ora-Blend}{4\ ml\ mixture} \times \frac{5\ ml\ mixture}{1}$$

= 1.25 mL Ora-Blend

Calculating for Simple syrup

4 mL mixture → 3 mL Simple syrup

5 mL mixture → u

$$u = \frac{3\ mL\ Simple\ syrup}{4\ mL\ mixture} \times \frac{5\ mL\ mixture}{1}$$

= 3.75 mL Simple syrup

Therefore, every 5 mL of the mixture contains 1.25 mL of Ora-Blend and 3.75 mL of Simple syrup.

$$1.25 + 3.75 = 5\ mL$$

Example 3.8

Due to the nature of the jobs, a pharmaceutical company has the target of employing women and men at the ratio of 2:3. Their target is to engage 600 employees in the current year. At present, they have employed 200 women and 200 men. How many more women and how many more men do they need to employ to meet both their numbers and ratio target?

Solution

Women   oo ⎤
         ⎥ Total 5 employees
Men   ●●● ⎦

Therefore:

For every 5 employees, there are 2 women.

For every 5 employees, there are 3 men.

$$5 \text{ total employees} \rightarrow 2 \text{ women employees}$$
$$5 \text{ total employees} \rightarrow 3 \text{ men employees}$$

Calculating for women employees

$$5 \text{ total employees} \rightarrow 2 \text{ women employees}$$
$$600 \text{ total employees} \rightarrow u$$

$$u = \frac{2 \text{ women employees}}{5 \text{ total employees}} \times \frac{600 \text{ total employees}}{1}$$

$$= 240 \text{ women employees}$$

Since they have already employed 200, they have 40 more women employees to engage.

Calculating for male employees

$$5 \text{ total employees} \rightarrow 3 \text{ men employees}$$
$$600 \text{ total employees} \rightarrow u$$

$$u = \frac{3 \text{ men employees}}{5 \text{ total employees}} \times \frac{600 \text{ total employees}}{1}$$

$$= 360 \text{ employees}$$

Since they have already employed 200 men, they still need 160 men employees to meet their target.

Example 3.9

The physician ordered the following prescription:

Rx

Mix Bactroban ointment: Cyclocort ointment (3:5).

Apply approximately 5 g to the affected area as needed.

Make 200 g.

How many grams of Bactroban and Cyclocort are needed to be mixed?

Solution

$$
\left.
\begin{array}{l}
\text{Bactroban} \quad \bullet\bullet\bullet \, 3\,g \\[2mm]
\text{Cyclocort} \quad \circ\circ\circ\circ\circ \, 5\,g
\end{array}
\right\} \text{Total 8 g}
$$

8 g mixture → 3 g Bactroban

8 g mixture → 5 g Cyclocort

Calculating for Bactroban

8 g mixture → 3 g Bactroban

200 g mixture → u

$$u = \frac{3\ g\ Bactroban}{8\ g\ mixture} \times \frac{200\ g\ mixture}{1}$$

= 75 g Bactroban

Calculating for Cyclocort

8 g mixture → 5 g Cyclocort

200 g mixture → u

$$u = \frac{5\ g\ Cyclocort}{8\ g\ mixure} \times \frac{200\ g\ mixture}{1}$$

= 125 g Cyclocort

200 g mixture = 75 g Bactroban + 125 g Cyclocort

Example 3.10

In the example 3.9 above, what amount of Bactroban and Cyclocort (in grams) is contained per application of the mixture?

Solution

5 grams is the quantity per application.

Calculating for Bactroban present (per 5 gram application only)

$$8 \text{ g mixture} \rightarrow 3 \text{ g Bactroban}$$

$$5 \text{ g mixture (application only)} \rightarrow u$$

$$u = \frac{3 \text{ g Bactroban}}{8 \text{ g mixture}} \times \frac{5 \text{ g mixture}}{1}$$

$$= 1.875 \text{ g}$$

Calculating for Cyclocort present (per 5 gram application only)

$$8 \text{ g mixture} \rightarrow 5 \text{ g Cyclocort}$$

$$5 \text{ g mixture (application only)} \rightarrow u$$

$$u = \frac{5 \text{ g Cyclocort}}{8 \text{ g mixture}} \times \frac{5 \text{ g mixture}}{1}$$

$$= 3.125 \text{ g Cyclocort per application}$$

Therefore, each 5 g of application mixture contains 1.875 g Bactroban and 3.125 g Cyclocort.

Introduction to Percentages

The percent is a very essential part of pharmaceutical calculations. The pharmacist or pharmacy technician/assistant encounters it frequently, and it is commonly used as an excellent means of expressing the amount of an active or inactive ingredient in a pharmaceutical preparation.

The term *percent* and the sign (%) that accompanies it means "per 100" or by the hundred. It is a ratio of a sort (part of a whole) where the whole is 100. For example, 5:100 = 5% = 5 out of every 100.

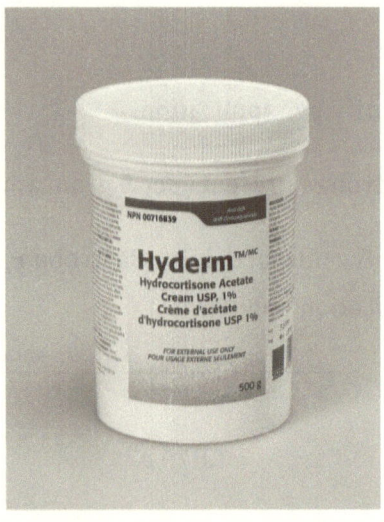

FIGURE 3.2 *The Taro-Hyderm Cream 1%:* One percent means 1 per 100. For every 100 gram of this formulation, there is 1 gram of the active ingredient, hydrocortisone. (Courtesy of Taro pharmaceuticals)

If we say that 40% of all the pharmacists in Calgary have Additional Prescribing Authorization (APA), it means that out of every 100 pharmacists in Calgary, 40 have APA. This statement looks like that of proportion, which can be represented as:

100 pharmacists in Calgary → 40 APA pharmacists

With this expression, given the total number of pharmacists in Calgary, it will be an easy task to calculate the expected number of APA pharmacists. If we also know the number of APA pharmacists, it will also be an easy task to determine the total number of pharmacists in Calgary using simple proportion principles.

If it is said that 30% of the entire student population of a particular university of pharmacy speak more than one language, it means that out of every hundred student in that university, 30 students speak more than one language. However, this does not mean that the entire population of the university is 100. It means that if we are able to "compress" the population of the university to 100, 30 students speak more than one language.

Percentage is somewhat always an abstract quantity and therefore can be variously applied to different concepts. Percentage tries to "shrink" the quantity in consideration to 100, giving us a line of proportion from which other unknown quantities can be calculated. Percentage is yet another type of fraction with a seemingly unexpressed denominator that is conventionally understood to represent 100.

$$30\% = \frac{30}{100} = 0.3$$

If the concentration of diclofenac in diclofenac ointment is 8%, it means that every 100 g of the said ointment (formulation) must contain only 8 g of diclofenac (the active ingredient). This can also be represented proportionally, thus

$$100 \text{ g ointment} \rightarrow 8 \text{ g diclofenac}$$
$$8 \text{ g diclofenac} \rightarrow 100 \text{ g ointment}$$

From the above expression, we can actually calculate the expected quantity (weight) of diclofenac if we know the amount of the ointment in question. We can also calculate the amount of the ointment we can make with an available amount of diclofenac powder (active ingredient).

Example 3.11

In a certain family, 30% of their income is spent on medication. If the income of the family is $48,000 a year, how much of the income is expected to be spent on medication for that year?

Solution

With 30% being spent on medication, it means that for every $100 of the family's income, $30 will be spent on medication and $70 on other things.

This can be represented proportionally, thus

$100 income → $30 medication

or

$30 medication → $100 income

Because we are looking for the amount spent on medication, the first line of expression will be more relevant in solving this problem because it has the medication expense part on the right.

$100 income → $30 medication

$48,000 income → u

$$u = \frac{\$30\ medication}{\$100\ income} \times \frac{\$48,000\ income}{1}$$

= $14,400 spent on medication

Therefore, from the income of $48,000, around $14,400 will be spent on drugs if the 30% expense on medication is correct. Realize that we are not interested in the remaining 70% because we do not know exactly what this family does with it.

Example 3.12

The pharmacist wants to make a 3% hydrocortisone cream in Glaxal base. How many grams of hydrocortisone powder are required to make 160 g of the cream?

Solution

3% hydrocortisone (HC) cream means that every 100 g of the final formulation (cream) must contain 3 g of pure HC powder.

We can represent this information as

$$100 \text{ g final cream} \rightarrow 3 \text{ g HC}$$

or

$$3 \text{ g HC} \rightarrow 100 \text{ g final cream}$$

Because we are looking for the amount of pure hydrocortisone, we will use the first expression.

$$100 \text{ g final cream} \rightarrow 3 \text{ g HC}$$
$$160 \text{ g final cream} \rightarrow u$$

$$u = \frac{3 \ g \ HC}{100 \ g \ final \ cream} \times \frac{160 \ g \ final \ cream}{1}$$

$$= 4.8 \text{ g}$$

Therefore, if 3 g HC are needed to make 100 g of the HC cream in Glaxal base (i.e., 3%), 4.8 g HC will be needed to make 160 g of same cream.

Example 3.13

A pharmacy bought some drugs at the cost of $12.89 and sold the drug at the price of $15.23. What is the percentage profit?

Solution

Profit made in the transaction is $15.23 – $12.89 = $2.34

The real question is, if the pharmacy made a profit of $2.34 in a product that cost $12.89, how much profit will the pharmacy make if the cost price was $100? (*Percent* means per 100.)

We can represent the proportion, thus

$$\$12.89 \text{ cost} \rightarrow \$2.34 \text{ profit}$$

$$\$100 \text{ cost} \rightarrow u$$

$$u = \frac{\$2.34 \; profit}{\$12.89 \; cost} \times \frac{\$100 \; cost}{1}$$

= $18.15 profit from every $100 cost

The last statement above defines percentage in its simplest form (amount per 100). The 18.15 will be taken as the percentage profit.

So the percentage profit is 18.15%

Note: It will be wise to attach identification to the figures, such as *cost* and *profit*. This enables them to be tracked, as both ends of the line of proportion are also sharing the unit $.

Example 3.14

A pharmacy bought some special cough syrup at the cost of $41.82. Due to poor demand and short expiry date, the pharmacy had to quickly sell the cough syrup below cost price for $38.45. What is the percentage loss sustained by the pharmacy on the cough syrup transaction?

Solution

The loss on the transaction is $41.82 – $38.45 = $3.37

The percentage loss is actually the loss per $100 cost of transaction. That is to say, if the pharmacy incurred the loss of $3.37 through a transaction of $41.82, how much loss would they have incurred if the transaction cost was $100?

$$\$41.82 \text{ cost} \rightarrow \$3.37 \text{ loss}$$

$$\$100 \text{ cost} \rightarrow u$$

$$u = \frac{\$3.37 \text{ loss}}{\$41.82 \text{ cost}} \times \frac{\$100 \text{ cost}}{1}$$

=$8.06 loss per $100 cost.

This statement defines percentage loss in its simplified form.

So the percentage loss is 8.06%

Example 3.15

A pharmacy wants to increase the selling price of a product by 40%. How much will the selling price of an item be if the original selling price is $120?

Solution

Increasing price by 40% means that for every $100 original selling price, $40 is added on top of the original price. This question is therefore seeking to ask, "If $40 extra is added for every $100 original price, how much will be the extra added on $120?"

$100 original price → $40 added

$120 original price → u

$$u = \frac{\$40 \text{ added}}{\$100 \text{ original price}} \times \frac{\$120 \text{ original price}}{1}$$

= $48 added on top of the original price

The new selling price will be original price + extra cost added.

$120 + $48 = $168 (new price)

Alternately we can say that for every $100 original price, new selling price will be $140 (40%).

That is,

$$\text{\$100 original price} \rightarrow \text{\$140 new price}$$
$$\text{\$120 original price} \rightarrow u$$

$$u = \frac{\$140 \; new \; price}{\$100 \; original \; price} \times \frac{\$120 \; original \; price}{1}$$

$$= \$168 \text{ new price}$$

Example 3.16

The pharmacy's wholesale dealer promises to give the pharmacy a discount of 15% if the pharmacy pays its debt within two weeks. If the pharmacy has a debt of $8,350 and pays the debt within two weeks, how much will the pharmacy be paying to the distributor, and how much will the pharmacy save by the smart move?

Solution

First of all, 15% discount means that for every debt of $100, there will be a discount of $15.

When we get the discount amount, we will then subtract it from the total bill. The result will be what the pharmacy will ultimately pay.

So using our proportion, every $100 attracts a discount of $15. (This is the meaning of 15% *discount*.)

Hence,

$$\text{\$100 debt} \rightarrow \text{\$15 discount}$$
$$\text{\$8,350 debt} \rightarrow u$$

$$u = \frac{\$15 \; discount}{\$100 \; debt} \times \frac{\$8,350 \; debt}{1}$$

$$= \$1,252.50 \text{ discount}$$

This is the discount that will be given for a debt of $8,350.

Therefore, the pharmacy will end up paying

$$\$8,350 - \$1,252.50 = \$7,097.50$$

The pharmacy will save an amount equivalent to the discount given, which is $1,252.50.

Example 3.17

A pharmacy is having a big sale, giving 25% off the label price of every cough and cold preparation on the shelf. Calculate the selling price of 1 box of Tylenol cough and cold if the labeled price is $28.37.

Solution

The meaning of 25% off is that if the product's labeled price is $100, the patient will get a discount of $25.

$$\$100 \text{ selling price} \rightarrow \$25 \text{ discount}$$
$$\$28.37 \text{ selling price} \rightarrow u$$

$$u = \frac{\$25 \; discount}{\$100 \; selling \; price} \times \frac{\$28.37 \text{ selling price}}{1}$$

$$= \$7.09 \text{ discount}$$

Note that this is just the discount and not what the patient will pay. So what the patient pays will be

$$\text{Total labeled price} - \text{discount}$$
$$\$28.37 - \$7.09 = \$21.28$$

Alternatively, we can say that 25% discount means that for every labeled price of $100, the patient is given a cash back of $25, so the patient actually pays $75.

That is,

$$\$100 \text{ labeled price} \rightarrow \$75 \text{ patient's payment}$$

$$\$28.37 \text{ labeled price} \rightarrow u$$

$$u = \frac{\$75 \text{ patient's payment}}{\$100 \text{ labeled price}} \times \frac{\$28.37 \text{ labeled price}}{1}$$

= $21.28 (the amount the patient will ultimately pay instead of the labeled price of $28.37)

Example 3.18

Your pharmacy received a shipment order of 250 blood pressure monitors. About 18% of the blood pressure monitors that were shipped were faulty and must be returned. How many of the blood pressure monitors will be returned?

Solution

That 18% were faulty means that out of every 100 blood pressure monitors, 18 were faulty. So we can say

$$100 \text{ BP monitors} \rightarrow 18 \text{ faulty}$$

$$250 \text{ BP monitors} \rightarrow u$$

$$u = \frac{18 \text{ faulty}}{100 \text{ BP monitors}} \times \frac{250 \text{ BP monitors}}{1}$$

$$= 45 \text{ BP monitors}$$

Therefore, 45 BP monitors are faulty and must be returned to the supplier.

Example 3.19

For a certain product in the pharmacy, the pharmacy is giving 19% discount on its sale while the manufacturer is giving a 6.5% discount to the pharmacy for the entire product sold. If the pharmacy sells a total of $980 worth of the product, how much will the pharmacy lose after the manufacturer's discount of 6.5%?

Solution

This problem can be approached in different ways:

Net discount = pharmacy's discount – company's discount.

$$19 - 6.5 = 12.5\%$$

Realize this discount is a negative one as far as the pharmacy is concerned.

The negative 12.5% means that for every $100 sold on the product, the pharmacy loses $12.5 on discount.

$100 sale → $12.5 discount

$980 sale → u

$$u = \frac{\$12.5 \text{ discount}}{\$100 \text{ sale}} \times \frac{\$980 \text{ sale}}{1}$$

= $122.50 total discount and loss to the pharmacy

Alternatively, we can calculate how much the company pays back to the pharmacy on one hand, calculate how much the pharmacy pays back to customers on the other hand, and subtract the two, thus getting the pharmacy's net loss in the transaction.

$100 sold → $6.5 (company's payment to pharmacy)

$980 sold → u

$$u = \frac{\$6.5 \text{ (company's payment to pharmacy)}}{\$100 \text{ sold}} \times \frac{\$980 \text{ sold}}{1}$$

= $63.70 (company's payment to the pharmacy)

The amount the pharmacy will pay to customers (19%)

$100 sold → $19 (pharmacy's payment to customers)

$980 sold → u

$$u = \frac{\$19\ (\text{pharmacy's payment to customers})}{\$100\ \text{sold}} \times \frac{\$980\ \text{sold}}{1}$$

$$= \$186.20$$

So $63.70 comes to the pharmacy, and $186.20 goes out. The net amount going out is

$$\$186.20 - \$63.70 = \$122.50$$

Example 3.20

As a way of promotion of the pharmacy's business, all customers filling their prescriptions in the pharmacy for the first time will receive a discount of 8.5%. What will be the dollar amount lost by the pharmacy if all new customers filling their prescription for the very first time brought in total business of $22,090?

Solution

Receiving a discount of 8.5% means that new customers will receive $8.5 for every $100 revenue. The question is therefore asking this:

If new customers receive $8.5 for every $100 revenue, how much total will customers filling their prescription for the first time receive if the total pharmacy revenue for the day is $22,090?

$$\$100\ \text{spent} → \$8.5\ \text{discount}$$

$$\$22{,}090\ \text{spent} → u$$

$$u = \frac{\$8.5\ \text{discount}}{\$100\ \text{spent}} \times \frac{\$22{,}090\ \text{spent}}{1}$$

$$= \$1{,}877.65\ \text{given out as discount at the end of the day.}$$

Example 3.21

By selling a cough syrup for $9.28 a pharmacist makes a 25% profit. What could have be the cost price of the cough syrup?

Solution

This is a little out of the ordinary, but simple logic will get us going toward the solution to this problem. A profit of 25% means that if the cost price of the product is $100, the product is sold with a profit of $25, which means the selling price would be $125. Now we are looking for the cost price given the selling price. We therefore need to arrange our line of proportion such that the cost price will be at the right-hand side of the equation. Thus

$$\$125 \text{ selling price} \rightarrow 100 \text{ cost price}$$
$$\$9.28 \text{ selling price} \rightarrow u$$

$$u = \frac{\$100 \text{ cost price}}{\$125 \text{ selling price}} \times \frac{\$9.28 \text{ selling price}}{1}$$

$$= \$7.43 \text{ cost price}$$

So the cost price of the item was $7.43.

Example 3.22

After the pharmacy sold OTC lice preparation, Nix, for $16.25, it was confirmed that they absorbed a 13% loss. What must have been the cost price of the OTC lice preparation?

Solution

A loss of 13% means that if the cost price of the product is $100, the product is sold with a loss of $13, which means the selling price will be ($100–$13 =) $87. Now we are looking for the cost price given the selling price. We therefore need to arrange our line of proportion such that the cost price will be at the right-hand side of the equation. Thus,

$87 selling price → $100 cost price

$16.25 selling price → u

$$u = \frac{\$100 \text{ cost price}}{\$87 \text{ selling price}} \times \frac{\$16.25 \text{ selling price}}{1}$$

$$= \$18.68 \text{ cost price}$$

Chapter 3 Practice Questions

Ratio

1. The physician requested that 150 grams of Viaderm KC be mixed with a certain amount (in grams) of Fucidin cream to make a 3:5 mixture. What is the amount of Fucidin cream that was to be mixed with 150 grams of Viaderm KC?

2. The ratio of men and women during a pharmacists' educational seminar was 3:4. If the number of men present at the seminar was 21, how many women will be expected to be present at the seminar?

3. Betaderm cream, 30 grams, is mixed with Emo-Cort cream, 50 grams. What amount of Emo-Cort will be present in 1 gram of the mixture?

4. You receive the following order:

    Rx

    Deep Heat + Vaseline 2:3

    Apply to both knees TID

    Make 120g

    How many grams of Deep Heat and Vaseline will be mixed to satisfy both the ratio and the quantity prescribed?

5. Distilled water was mixed solely with ethanol such that every 8 mL of the resulting mixture contains 3 mL of ethanol. What is the ratio of distilled water: ethanol in the mixture?

6. You receive the following order:

Rx

Vaseline : Glaxal base (2:5)

Sig: Apply to eczema

Make 200 g

How many grams of Vaseline will be needed to make the compound?

7. A pharmacist mixed 15 g of Hyderm cream and 60 g of nystatin cream together to make a homogeneous blend.

(a) What is the ratio of Hyderm : nystatin in the final mix?

(b) What amount of Hyderm will be present in 15 grams of the mixture?

8. If 40 mL of simple syrup is mixed with 50 mL of Ora-Blend, what is the combination ratio? How many milliliters of simple syrup are present in each milliliter of the mixture?

9. For the treatment of eczema, a physician likes to use a special formulation of topical emollients that is a combination of Aquaphor and CeraVe at a ratio of 3:8. To make 220 g of the emollient, how many grams of Aquaphor and CeraVe will be needed?

10. Alcohol and distilled water are mixed together in a ratio of 4:5. How many milliliters of alcohol will be needed to make 180 mL of the mixture?

11. Two solutions, A and B, are combined in a 3:1 ratio to make a custom compounded solution. How many milliliters of each is required to make 200 mL of this mixture?

12. Mixed together are 30 g of Fucidin H and 45 g of Vaseline.

    (a) What is the ratio of Fucidin H : Vaseline in the final mixture?

    (b) What amount of Vaseline will be present in 300 g of the mixture?

13. A special compound requires two ingredients, A and B, to be mixed at a ratio of A:B = 4:7. What amount of the final product can be made with only 12 g of A?

14. You received the following prescription:

    Rx

    Mix Hyderm: Cortoderm in the ratio of 2:3

    How many grams of Cortoderm will be needed
    to make 50 grams of the mixture?

15. You receive the following order:

    Rx

    Dermovate cream: desonide cream (2:3)

    Sig: Apply 5 g to affected area as needed

    Make 200 g

    How many grams of Dermovate cream and desonide
    cream will be present per application of the mixture?

16. The physician ordered the pharmacy to mix perichlor mouth rinse and Tantum liquid at a ratio of 1:4. How many milliliters of each liquid will be required to make 200 mL of the mixture?

17. Cortoderm and Hyderm are mixed together such that every 5 g of the mixture contains 1 g of Cortoderm. What is the ratio of Cortoderm : Hyderm in the mixture?

18. A pharmacist set out to make 500 g of a 2:3 mixture of Canesten cream and Emo-Cort cream. Before the compounding started, he discovered he only has 1 tube of Canesten cream (30 grams) but enough Emo-Cort cream. What is the maximum quantity of the mixture he can make to satisfy the ratio?

19. The prescription authorizes the pharmacist to mix Uremol with Betaderm at the ratio of 4:3. How much of the final mixture can be obtained from 48 g of Uremol?

20. A pharmacist sets out to make his own customized oral vehicle by mixing Ora-Blend and simple syrup at the ratio of 5:3. How many milliliters of Ora-Blend will be needed to make 160 mL of the customized oral?

21. A physician wants the pharmacist to mix clotrimazole cream and nystatin cream at the ratio of 3:2 for a baby's diaper rash. How much of the final mixture can be made using 45 g of the clotrimazole cream?

22. In a certain college where pharmacy technicians are trained, the population of male students is 1.5 times the number of female students.

(a) (a) Expressed as whole numbers without decimals, what is the ratio of male:female students in the college?

(b) (b) If the total population of the college is 300, how many students are male?

23. To treat certain kinds of eczema, the pharmacist normally mixes Cortoderm + Emo-Cort in a ratio of 4:5. How many grams of each will be required to make 220 pounds of the mixture?

24. To make a better-tasting oral suspension vehicle, the physician requires the pharmacist to mix Ora-Sweet and simple syrup at the ratio of 4:1. How many milliliters of the mixture can be achieved using 100 mL of the Ora-Sweet?

25. You receive the following prescription:

Rx

Mix Nyaderm cream : clotrimazole cream (7:3)

Apply to diaper rash TID and QHS

How many grams of clotrimazole are needed to make 200 g of the mixture?

Percentages

26. By selling a product at the price of $8, the pharmacy incurred a 20% loss. What could have been the cost price?

27. The pharmacy's markup on OTC Tylenol 1 is 35%. If the cost price of one bottle is $4.95, how much will the pharmacy sell to satisfy the markup?

28. Your wholesale dealer promises to give a discount of 20% if your debt of $23,890 is paid within one week. How much will you expect to receive back from your wholesale dealer if you pay that bill within one week?

29. A pharmacy bought some disposable syringes at the cost of $18.92 and sold them at the price of $20.52. What is the percentage profit?

30. A pharmacy planned to increase the price of an item by 25%. If the original price is $49.98, what will be the new selling price?

31. In a certain chain pharmacy, 20% of all the pharmacist employees are internationally trained. If there is a total of 900 pharmacist employees of the chain pharmacy, how many are internationally trained?

32. By selling a product for $86.40, a pharmacy makes a 70% profit. What must have been the cost price of the product?

33. A pharmacy technician just discovered that the dress she bought from Walmart for $9 was not the right size. She sold it on kijiji.ca for $5. What is the percentage loss on the transaction?

34. A pharmacy sells its cough syrup with codeine using a markup of 30%. If a patient paid $26 for the cough syrup, what was the cost price of the cough syrup?

35. A pharmacist made a 10% menthol ointment in Vaseline. If the total quantity of the ointment made is 180g, how many grams of menthol is contained in there?

36. A certain cream is said to contain 10% of the active ingredient. What is the ratio of active : inactive ingredients in the cream?

37. A pharmacy intends to make a 40% profit on an item that was bought for $80. To achieve this, at what price must the pharmacy sell the item?

38. In a certain pharmacy, 6% of their total revenue on Tuesdays goes to the golf club support fund. If the pharmacy made a total revenue of $15,825 on one Tuesday, how much will be sent to the gulf club support fund?

39. The physician ordered a mixture of Nyaderm and Hyderm at the ratio of 1:4. What is the percentage of Nyaderm in the combination?

40. A pharmacy bought some drugs from McKesson for $2,380. Suddenly there was a price reduction, and the pharmacy dispensed them for $1,982. What is the percentage loss?

41. A pharmacy gives 6% of their annual profit to the Salvation Army. If their target for the year is to give $24,000 to Salvation Army, what will be their target profit for the year?

42. A pharmacist told you he made a 15% loss by selling a blood pressure monitor for $90. What must have been the cost price?

43. About 5% of the employees of a company smoke cigarettes. If the company currently has 13 employees that are smokers, how many employees does the company have?

44. A certain pharmacy technician spends 3% of his total earnings on gas commuting to work. If his total earnings for 2016 were $28,595, how much was spent on gas commuting to work?

45. The CEO of a pharmacy chain declared a loss of 18% for the fiscal year. According to the CEO, it was confirmed that the company lost $22,000. What was the total revenue of the company for the said fiscal year?

46. A certain company gives 15% of the yearly revenue to charity. How much is expected to go to charity in that year if the total revenue of the pharmacy is $96,400 in a year?

47. A pharmacy technician bought a car for $28,000 and finally resold it for $28,500. What is the percentage profit?

48. Your pharmacy is offering 25% discount on first aid products on the shelf. If the original price of hydrogen peroxide is $8.82, how much will a customer pay with the 25% discount?

49. If you spend 2% of your income on groceries, 5% on gas, and 4% on travels, how much will your total expense on groceries, gas, and travels in a year be if your total income for that year is $52,800?

50. By selling a product for $120, the merchant made a 20% profit. What do you think is the cost price of the item?

You received the following order to prepare this topical ointment:

Rx

Menthol 5%, cyclobenzaprine 12%,
diclofenac 3% in Aquaphor

Make 400 grams

What is the ratio of the inactive base to the entire formulation?

Answers to Chapter 3
Practice Questions

1. 250 g Fucidin cream
2. 28 women
3. 0.625 g Emo-Cort
4. 48 g Deep Heat, 72 g Vaseline
5. 5:3 (Distilled water:ethanol)
6. 57.143 g Vaseline
7. (a) 1:4 (Hyderm:nystatin)
   (b) 3 g Hyderm
8. 4:5 (Simple syrup:Ora-Blend)
   0.4444 mL simple syrup
9. 60 g Aquaphor
   160 g CeraVe
10. 80 mL alcohol
11. 150 mL solution A, 50 mL solution B
12. (a) 2:3 (Fucidin H:Vaseline)
    (b) 180 g Vaseline
13. 33 g of A
14. 30 g Cortoderm
15. 2 g Dermovate cream, 3 g desonide cream
16. 40 mL perichlor, 160 mL Tantum
17. 1:4 (Cortoderm:Hyderm)
18. 75 g mixture
19. 84 g mixture
20. 100 mL Ora-Blend
21. 75 g mixture
22. (a) 3:2 (male:female)
    (b) 180 males
23. 44,444.44 g Cortoderm
    55,555.56 g Emo-Cort
24. 125 mL mixture
25. 60 g clotrimazole
26. $10

27. $6.68
28. $4,778
29. 8.46%
30. $62.48
31. 180 employees
32. $50.82
33. 44.44%
34. 20%
35. 18 g
36. 1:9 (active ingredient: inactive ingredient)
37. $112
38. $949.5
39. 20%
40. 16.72%
41. $400,000
42. $105.88
43. 260 employees
44. $857.85
45. $122,222.22
46. $14,460
47. 1.79%
48. $6.62
49. $5,808
50. $100

Solution to Star Question

First we need to know the amount of each ingredient present in the entire formulation.

Amount of menthol

$$100 \text{ g formulation} \rightarrow 5 \text{ g menthol}$$
$$400 \text{ g of formulation} \rightarrow u$$
$$u = \frac{5 \text{ g menthol}}{100 \text{ g formulation}} \times \frac{400 \text{ g formulation}}{1}$$
$$= 20 \text{ g of menthol}$$

Amount of cyclobenzaprine

$$100 \text{ g formulation} \rightarrow 12 \text{ g cyclobenzaprine}$$
$$400 \text{ g of formulation} \rightarrow u$$
$$u = \frac{12 \text{ g cyclobenzaprine}}{100 \text{ g formulation}} \times \frac{400 \text{ g formulation}}{1}$$
$$= 48 \text{ g}$$

Amount of diclofenac

$$100 \text{ g formulation} \rightarrow 3 \text{ g diclofenac}$$
$$400 \text{ g of formulation} \rightarrow u$$
$$u = \frac{3 \text{ g diclofenac}}{100 \text{ g formulation}} \times \frac{400 \text{ g formulation}}{1}$$
$$= 12 \text{ g diclofenac}$$

Total amount of active ingredient in the 400 g of the formulation is

$$20 \text{ g} + 48 \text{ g} + 12 \text{ g}$$
$$= 80 \text{ g}$$

The amount of the base (inactive ingredient) is

Amount of total formulation – amount of active ingredients
$$= 400 \text{ g} - 80 \text{ g}$$
$$= 320 \text{ g of inactive base (Aquaphor)}$$

Ratio of inactive base to the entire formulation is

$$= 320 \text{ g} : 400 \text{ g}$$
$$= 4 : 5$$

CHAPTER 4

Expressions of Concentration of Pharmaceutical Formulations

Objectives

At the end of this chapter, students should be able to do the following:

- Demonstrate understanding of the various ways the concentration of active ingredients are expressed in a formulation
- Calculate the percentage concentration, the ratio concentration, and the fractional concentration of a formulation
- Perform and accomplish simple calculations involving concentration expressions
- Interconvert one form of concentration expression to the other

Introduction

From the time of the apothecaries to the present day, medications are rarely administered as pure drug substances containing only the drug molecules. Consumable medications are products of formulation. Formulation is the process whereby pure drug molecules are mixed with some inactive excipients (such as bases, sweeteners, lubricants, suspending agents, flavors, etc.) at a very defined proportion to make pharmaceutical formulations like suspensions, tablets, capsules, liniments, ointments, creams, pastes, elixirs, and the like.

Consumable medication = pure drug
substance + inactive ingredients

Therefore, most pharmaceutical formulations contain both the active ingredient (the pure drug molecules) and the inactive ingredient(s). The proportion of the *active ingredient* in a pharmaceutical formulation compared to that of a definite (or defined) portion of the *formulation* is referred to as the concentration of the drug in the formulation. In pharmacy, the concentration of the active ingredient in a formulation can be expressed in various ways. Proper understanding of these expressions of concentrations is vital to accurate calculations involving concentrations.

The various ways of expressing the concentration of pharmaceutical formulations are:

- ✓ Percentage concentration
- ✓ Ratio concentration
- ✓ Freestyle/conventional/fractional concentration

Percentage Concentrations

Just as previously discussed in the chapter on percentages, percent (%) means "per 100." A 5% concentration means that 5 parts of the active ingredient are present in 100 parts of the formulation. A 7.5% concentration means that 7.5 units of the active ingredient are present in 100 units of the formulation.

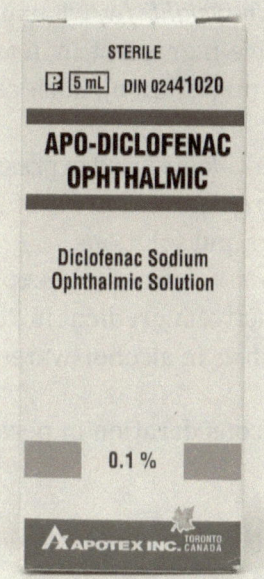

FIGURE 4.1 *Apo-Diclofenac Ophthalmic 0.1%:* The percentage strength of
0.1% means that 0.1 gram (100 mg) of the active ingredient (diclofenac) is
contained in every 100 mL of the formulation. (Courtesy Apotex)

By Definition

Conventionally, the unit of the active ingredient is usually in grams
(g). It can also be expressed in milliliters for those drug molecules that
are liquid in their very pure form.

The unit of formulation is measured in

- milliliters, if the final formulation is a liquid preparation, or
- gram, if the final formulation is solid or semisolid preparation.

In pharmaceutical calculations, an expressed percentage concentration
can be any of the following:

➢ weight–weight (% w/w)
➢ weight–volume (% w/v)
➢ volume–volume (% v/v)

- *Percent weight-in-weight (w/w)* expresses the number of *grams* of an active ingredient in *100 g* of solid or semisolid formulation (or preparation), such as in creams, ointments, and the like.
- *Percent weight-in-volume (w/v)* expresses the amount in *grams* of the active ingredient in *100 mL* of liquid preparation, such as in suspensions and solutions.
- *Percent volume-in-volume (v/v)* expresses the number of *milliliters* of an active ingredient in *100 mL* of the final liquid preparation, such as in alcohol/water solution.

Note: The two units of consideration in percentage expressions are *grams* and *milliliters*.

X% is either of the following:

- *X g* active ingredient in *100 g* of solid/semisolid preparation (w/w)
- *X g* active ingredient in *100 mL* of liquid preparation (w/v)
- *X mL* of active ingredient in *100 mL* of liquid preparation (v/v)

Therefore, expressed percentage can be either w/v, w/w, or v/v only, depending on the nature of final formulation and the nature of active ingredient added.

The percentage concentration of liquid preparations is normally in w/v or v/v, and that of solid or semisolid preparations are usually in w/w.

An expressed percentage does not actually need to carry the suffix v/v, w/v, or w/w. The nature of the active ingredient and the form of the final formulation gives the clue.

The most commonly expressed percentage is w/v and w/w.

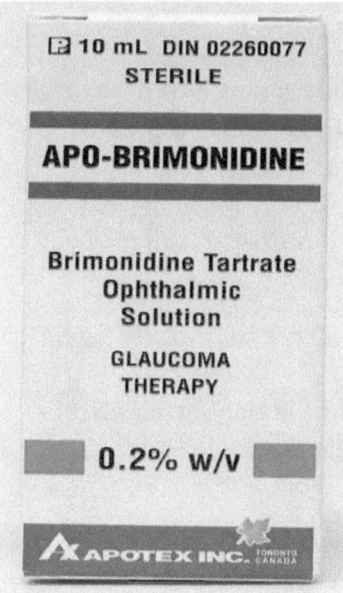

FIGURE 4.2 *Apo-Brimonidine 0.2%:* The strength of 0.2% means that every 100 mL of the formulation contains 0.2 gram (200 mg) of the pure active ingredient, brimonidine. (Courtesy Apotex)

Examples

A 5% suspension of enalapril means that every 100 mL of the suspension contains 5 g of the enalapril active drug (%w/v).

Similarly, a 3% atropine solution contains 3 g of atropine active drug in every 100 mL of the solution (%w/v).

A 10% diclofenac gel means that every 100 g of the final formulation (gel) contains 10 g of diclofenac active drug (%w/w).

A 70% alcohol solution means that every 100 mL of the solution contains 70 mL of pure liquid alcohol (%v/v).

Example 4.1

If 5 g of sodium nitrate is dissolved in 180 mL of water, what is the percentage strength of the resulting solution?

Solution

This question is actually asking us how many grams of sodium nitrate will be in 100 mL of the solution prepared. We can represent our information using proportion. Thus,

$$5 \text{ g NaNO}_3 \rightarrow 180 \text{ mL solution}$$

or

$$180 \text{ mL solution} \rightarrow 5 \text{ g NaNO}_3$$

Now we are looking for the amount of $NaNO_3$, so we will use the second expression because that expression has a $NaNO_3$ component to the right.

$$180 \text{ mL solution} \rightarrow 5 \text{ g NaNO}_3$$
$$100 \text{ mL solution} \rightarrow u$$

$$u = \frac{5 \text{ g NaNO}_3}{180 \text{ mL solution}} \times \frac{100 \text{ mL solution}}{1}$$

= 2.78 grams of $NaNO_3$ in every 100 mL of the solution

The statement above is a typical definition of the percentage strength of a solution. Hence, the percentage strength is 2.78%.

Example 4.2

How many grams of table salt will be required to make 300 mL of a 6% table salt solution?

Solution

The solution to this problem begins from understanding the term 6%. If the percentage concentration of the solution is 6%, it means that every 100 mL of that solution must contain 6 g of the table salt.

$$100 \text{ mL solution} \rightarrow 6 \text{ g table salt}$$

or

$$6 \text{ g table salt} \rightarrow 100 \text{ mL solution}$$

The question is seeking to ask: *If* 6 g of table salt is contained in 100 mL of the solution, how many grams of the table salt will be contained in 300 mL? We will use the first line of proportion statement (because the quantity of table salt is on the right).

$$100 \text{ mL solution} \rightarrow 6 \text{ g table salt}$$

$$300 \text{ mL solution} \rightarrow u$$

$$u = \frac{6 \text{ g table salt}}{100 \text{ mL solution}} \times \frac{300 \text{ mL solution}}{1}$$

$$= 18 \text{ g of table salt}$$

To make 300 mL of 6% table salt solution, I simply need to dissolve 18 g of table salt and make the volume up to 300 mL.

Example 4.3

How many grams of dextrose will be used in making the following prescription?

Rx

Dextrose solution 4% in distilled water

Sig: Use for infusion as directed.

Make 350 mL

Solution

The prescription above calls for a 4% dextrose solution. In pharmacy, 4% dextrose solution means only one thing: Each 100 mL of the solution must contain 4 g of the dextrose. The prescription above is authorizing the pharmacist to make 350 mL. In other words, the question is asking: If 4 g of dextrose is contained in 100 mL of solution, how many grams of dextrose will be contained in 350 mL?

Keeping the dextrose gram portion to the right, we write

$$100 \text{ mL solution} \rightarrow 4 \text{ g dextrose}$$
$$350 \text{ mL solution} \rightarrow u$$
$$u = \frac{4 \text{ g dextrose}}{100 \text{ mL solution}} \times \frac{350 \text{ mL solution}}{1}$$
$$= 14 \text{ g dextrose}$$

Dissolving 14 g of dextrose in distilled water and making the volume 350 mL will produce a 4% dextrose solution.

Example 4.4

How many grams of potassium permanganate should be used in preparing 1.5 pints of 4% potassium permanganate solution?

Solution

Having 4% potassium permanganate means that every 100 mL of the solution must contain 4 g of potassium permanganate. The question is therefore asking this: If 4 g of potassium permanganate is contained in 100 mL, how many grams of potassium permanganate will be contained in 1.5 pint?

$$1 \text{ pint} \rightarrow 480 \text{ mL}$$
$$1.5 \text{ pint} \rightarrow u$$
$$u = \frac{480 \text{ mL}}{1 \text{ pint}} \times \frac{1.5 \text{ pint}}{1}$$
$$= 720 \text{ mL}$$

Note: We need to convert the pint to milliliters because percentage concentration is the expression involving grams of the active ingredient and 100 *milliliters* of the preparation.

So we write our proportional relationship, keeping potassium permanganate to the right.

$$100 \text{ mL solution} \rightarrow 4 \text{ g KMnO}_4$$

$$720 \text{ mL solution} \rightarrow u$$

$$u = \frac{4 \text{ g KMnO}_4}{100 \text{ mL solution}} \times \frac{720 \text{ mL solution}}{1}$$

= 28.8 g potassium permanganate

Example 4.5

If a pharmacist set out to make an 8% suspension of prednisolone in Ora-Blend, how many milliliters of the suspension can be made from 24 g of pure prednisolone powder?

Solution

Making 8% suspension of prednisolone in Ora-Blend means that every 100 mL of the final formulation must contain 8 g prednisolone. The question is asking this: If 100 mL of suspension requires 8 g prednisolone, how many milliliters of the suspension will be made from 24 g of prednisolone?

Using our idea of proportion,

$$8 \text{ g prednisolone} \rightarrow 100 \text{ mL suspension}$$

$$24 \text{ g prednisolone} \rightarrow u$$

$$u = \frac{100 \text{ mL suspension}}{8 \text{ g prednisolone}} \times \frac{24 \text{ g prednisolone}}{1}$$

= 300 mL of prednisolone suspension

Example 4.6

When 20 g of hydrocortisone powder is mixed with 140 g of Glaxal base to form hydrocortisone cream, what is the percentage strength of the resulting cream?

Solution

Remember that this calculation is definitely w/w because both active and inactive components are quantified in grams.

% is expressed as g active ingredient per 100 g of *formulation*.

The formulation includes both active and inactive ingredients.

When 20 g hydrocortisone is mixed with 140 g of Glaxal base to make a formulation, the total weight of the formulation will be 20 + 140 = 160 g.

Thus we can say that 20 g hydrocortisone is contained in 160 g of final formulation.

Hence, the question is actually asking us how many grams of hydrocortisone will be contained in 100 g of the final formulation.

Using our proportion,

160 g formulation → 20 g hydrocortisone

100 g formulation → u

$$u = \frac{20 \text{ g hydrocortisone}}{160 \text{ g formulation}} \times \frac{100 \text{ g formulation}}{1}$$

= 12.5 g of hydrocortisone in 100 g formulation

This statement typically defines the percentage strength (g active ingredient in 100 g of the formulation [w/w]). Hence the percentage is 12.5%.

Note: It is wise to label our components when writing our proportion so they can be tracked. It can easily be observed that all the components in the proportion have gram as their unit. Merely attaching the unit *gram* will not be able to identify each component.

Example 4.7

What weight of a 12% cyclobenzaprine gel can be prepared using 6 g of the cyclobenzaprine active powder?

Solution

A 12% cyclobenzaprine gel is made such that 12 g of the active ingredient (cyclobenzaprine) is contained in every 100 g of the final formulation (gel). The question is asking this: If 100 g of the gel is made with 12 g of cyclobenzaprine, how many grams of the gel can be made using 6 g of the cyclobenzaprine powder?

Using our proportion,

$$12 \text{ g cyclobenzaprine} \rightarrow 100 \text{ g gel formulation}$$

$$(\text{Keeping formulation on the right})$$

$$6 \text{ g cyclobenzaprine} \rightarrow u$$

$$u = \frac{100 \text{ g gel formulation}}{12 \text{ g cyclobenzaprine}} \times \frac{6 \text{ g cyclobenzaprine}}{1}$$

$$= 50 \text{ g gel formulation}$$

Example 4.8

A pharmacist prepared a 2% clindamycin cream in Diffusimax. How many milligrams of the active ingredient (clindamycin) do you expect to be contained in 5 g of the final formulation?

Solution

Realize the active ingredient is clindamycin and the base (inactive ingredient) is the Diffusimax. Having 2% clindamycin means that every 100 g of the formulation contains only 2 g of the clindamycin active drug; the remainder is base.

Using our proportion,

100 g formulation → 2 g clindamycin

5 g formulation → u

$$u = \frac{2 \text{ g clindamycin}}{100 \text{ g formulation}} \times \frac{5 \text{ g formulation}}{1}$$

= 0.1 g of clindamycin

The answer is required in milligrams, so we need to convert the gram to its milligram equivalent.

But

1 g → 1,000 mg

0.1 g → u

$$u = \frac{1,000 \text{ mg}}{1 \text{ g}} \times \frac{0.1 \text{ g}}{1}$$

= 100 mg

Example 4.9

A cream on the pharmacy shelf is labeled Betaderm 0.1%. What amount of base (inactive ingredient) would you expect to be present in 80 g of the cream?

Solution

We can solve this problem in either of two of ways. We can calculate the amount of active ingredient (betamethasone) in 80 g of the cream then subtract this amount from 80 g formulation to get the amount of inactive ingredients (base) present.

100 g Betaderm cream → 0.1 g betamethasone

80 g Betaderm cream → u

$$u = \frac{0.1 \text{ g betamethasone}}{100 \text{ g Betaderm cream}} \times \frac{80 \text{ g Betaderm cream}}{1}$$

= 0.08 g of betamethasone

There is 0.08 g of active ingredient (betamethasone) present in 80 g of 0.1% Betaderm cream. The rest is inactive base.

That is,

$$80 - 0.08 = 79.92 \text{ g inactive base}$$

Otherwise, we can go directly:

Having 0.1% Betaderm cream means that every 100 g of the cream contains 0.1 g of betamethasone and the rest of the component is base (inactive). So inactive ingredient in 100 g is (100 g – 0.1 g) = 99.9 g base.

Using our proportion

$$100 \text{ g Betaderm cream} \rightarrow 99.9 \text{ g inactive base}$$

$$80 \text{ g Betaderm cream} \rightarrow u$$

$$u = \frac{99.9 \text{ g inactive base}}{100 \text{ g Betaderm cream}} \times \frac{80 \text{ g Betaderm cream}}{1}$$

$$= 79.92 \text{ g of inactive base}$$

Example 4.10

A prescription calls for a 4% lidocaine in Aquaphor (base), and 400 g were ordered. The pharmacist checks the compounding supply to discover that only 15 g of lidocaine and enough Aquaphor is available. The patient agrees that the pharmacist can make as much as possible depending on ingredient availability. How many grams of the ordered cream can the pharmacist make using the available lidocaine?

Solution

Making 4% lidocaine in Aquaphor (Aquaphor is the inactive ointment base) would require that every 100 g of the final formulation must contain 4 g of lidocaine. The question is therefore asking this: If 4 g of lidocaine powder can only make 100 g of the formulation (4%), what amount of formulation can 15 g of lidocaine make?

Using our proportion

$$4 \text{ g lidocaine} \rightarrow 100 \text{ g formulation}$$

$$15 \text{ g lidocaine} \rightarrow u$$

$$u = \frac{100 \text{ g formulation}}{4 \text{ g lidocaine}} \times \frac{15 \text{ g lidocaine}}{1}$$

$$= 375 \text{ g of the formulation}$$

The pharmacist can only make 375 g of the formulation given the available 15 g of the lidocaine powder.

Ratio Strength

The ratio strength is another way of expressing concentrations of especially weak formulations. The ratio strength is an extension of the percentage strength, but in the case of the ratio strength, effort is made to know the ratio of one part of the active ingredient compared to a defined amount of formulation. Ratio strength is merely another way of expressing the percentage strength of solution or liquid preparations, but in the case of the ratio strength, the active ingredient is always expressed as 1 g or 1 mL depending on the nature of the active ingredient.

A 2% solution of dextrose actually means 2 parts of dextrose:100 parts of solution = 2:100

Although this is a ratio of sort, in expressing ratio strength, it is conventional to reduce the active ingredient part to 1, so 2:100 = 1:50.

In ratio strength, the proportion ratio is modified such that the active ingredient assumes the value of 1 g or 1 mL.

When the ratio strength of a formulation is written as 1:50,000, the acceptable interpretation is as follows:

- For solid in liquid = 1 g of pure active ingredient in 50,000 mL of liquid preparation
- For liquid in liquid = 1 mL of pure active ingredient in 50,000 mL of liquid preparation
- For solid in solid = 1 g of pure active ingredient is 50,000 g of solid or semisolid preparation

Note: Just like in percentage strength, the units of measure for the active ingredient are grams (for solid active ingredients) and milliliters (for liquid active ingredient). The active ingredient must be expressed as 1 g or 1 mL compared to the amount in grams or milliliters of formulation that contains it.

Ratio strength is always expressed as

$$1:U$$

where 1 represents 1 g or 1 mL of pure active ingredient and U represents the corresponding parts of the formulation (in milliliters or grams) that contain the unit active ingredient.

Hence percentage strength can be converted to ratio strength and vice versa. If a concentration is in another unit of weight other than grams, it must be realized that the unit must be converted to grams first.

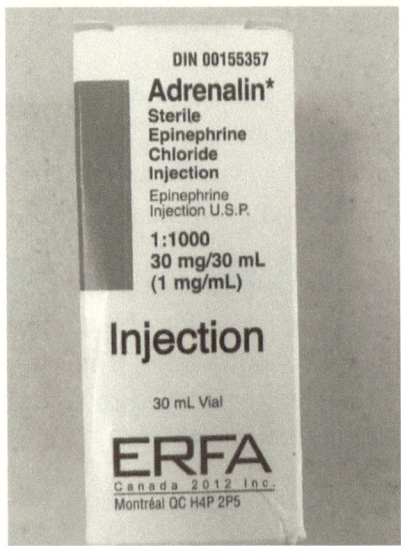

FIGURE 4.3 *Adrenaline Injection:* The adrenaline injectable solution with the Ratio Strength of 1:1000 means that 1 gram of pure adrenaline should be contained in every 1000 mL (1 Liter) of the solution. (Courtesy ERFA Canada Inc.)

Example 4.11

Convert 0.05% to ratio strength.

Solution

A 0.05% preparation contains 0.05 g of active ingredient in 100 parts of formulation. This question is seeking to find out what part of the formulation will contain just 1 g of the active ingredient.

Using our proportion,

0.05 g active ingredient → 100 parts formulation

1 g active ingredient → u

$$u = \frac{100 \text{ part formulation}}{0.05 \text{ g active ingredient}} \times \frac{1 \text{ g active ingredient}}{1}$$

= 2,000 parts of the formulation

It means that 1 g of the active ingredient will be contained in 2,000 parts of the formulation. This is a typical format for ratio strength. We can therefore comfortably express the ratio strength as 1:2,000.

So ratio strength = 1:2,000

Example 4.12

A pharmacist dissolved 2 g of a drug powder in enough distilled water to make 500 mL of solution. What is the ratio strength of the solution?

Solution

This question seeks to find out what part of the solution will contain just 1 gram of the drug.

So using our proportion,

2 g active ingredient → 500 mL solution

1 g active ingredient → u

$$u = \frac{500 \text{ mL solution}}{2 \text{ g active ingredient}} \times \frac{1 \text{ g ingredient}}{1}$$

= 250 mL solution

So 1 g of the active ingredient will be in 250 mL. Therefore, the ratio strength is 1:250.

Example 4.13

Pediatric prednisolone comes with a labeled strength of 1 mg in every 1 mL of solution. Express this concentration as ratio strength.

Solution

Ratio strength seeks to express the concentration of a formulation such that it is clearly evident what part of the formulation contains 1 g of the active ingredient.

If we say

$$1 \text{ mg} \rightarrow 1\text{mL}$$

$$1 \text{ g} \rightarrow \text{u},$$

the units on the left (mg and g) are not the same, so it will be wrong to proceed with the calculation as they are. Therefore, we need to convert the 1 mg to its gram equivalent.

$$1{,}000 \text{ mg} \rightarrow 1 \text{ g}$$

$$1 \text{ mg} \rightarrow \text{u}$$

$$\text{u} = \frac{1\,g}{1{,}000\,mg} \times \frac{1\,mg}{1}$$

$$= 0.001 \text{ g}$$

Continuing

$$0.001 \text{ g} \rightarrow 1 \text{ mL}$$

$$1 \text{ g} \rightarrow \text{u}$$

$$\text{u} = \frac{1\,mL}{0.001\,g} \times \frac{1\,g}{1}$$

$$= 1{,}000 \text{ mL}$$

So 1 gram of the active ingredient will be contained in 1,000 mL of the solution. Therefore, the ratio strength is 1:1,000.

Example 4.14

How can you express 1:5,000 ratio strength as percentage strength?

Solution

We already know what 1:5,000 ratio strength means. It implies that 1 g of active ingredient is contained in every 5,000 units of formulation. The question is actually asking us how many grams of the active ingredient will be in 100 units of the formulation (which defines the percentage strength).

Using our proportional relationship,

$$5{,}000 \text{ units of formulation} \rightarrow 1 \text{ g active ingredient}$$

$$100 \text{ unit of formulation (\%)} \rightarrow u$$

$$u = \frac{1 \text{ g active ingredient}}{5{,}000 \text{ units of formulation}} \times \frac{100 \text{ unit of formulation}}{1}$$

$$= 0.02 \text{ g of active ingredient in 100 parts of formulation.}$$

$$\text{This means } 0.02\%.$$

Example 4.15

A pharmacist crushed 4 tablets of 5 mg bisoprolol to make 200 mL of suspension with simple syrup oral vehicle. What is the ratio strength of the suspension?

Solution

The equivalent of 4 tablets of 5 mg bisoprolol is 4 × 5mg = 20 mg bisoprolol.

Therefore, technically, 20 mg of bisoprolol will be contained in the 200 mL of the suspension. The question is seeking to find out how many units of the formulation that will contain just 1 gram of bisoprolol.

We again use our proportion:

$$20 \text{ mg bisoprolol} \rightarrow 200 \text{ mL formulation}$$

$$1 \text{ g bisoprolol} \rightarrow u$$

Realize that the units on the left of the lines of proportion do not match, therefore the 20 mg must be converted to g or the 1 g must be converted to milligrams in order to proceed with the calculation.

Converting 20 mg to g

$$1{,}000 \text{ mg} \rightarrow 1 \text{ g}$$

$$20 \text{ mg} \rightarrow u$$

$$u = \frac{1\ g}{1{,}000\ mg} \times \frac{20\ mg}{1}$$

$$= 0.02 \text{ g}$$

Therefore, 20 mg is equivalent to 0.02 g. Now we can proceed!

Continuing with our calculation,

$$0.02 \text{ g bisoprolol} \rightarrow 200 \text{ mL formulation}$$

$$1 \text{ g bisoprolol} \rightarrow u$$

$$u = \frac{200\ mL\ formulation}{0.02\ g\ bisoprolol} \times \frac{1\ g\,bisoprolol}{1}$$

$$= 10{,}000 \text{ mL of formulation}$$

So 1 g of active ingredient (bisoprolol) will be contained in 10,000 mL of the formulation. Therefore, the ratio is 1:10,000.

Example 4.16

How many milligrams of amlodipine will be used in making 500 mL of 1:200 amlodipine suspensions?

Solution

First we focus on 1:200. A ratio of 1:200 means that 1 g of amlodipine is contained in 200 mL of the suspension. The question seeks to find out what amount of amlodipine (in milligrams) will be contained in 500 mL of the suspension.

So, using our proportion,

$$200 \text{ mL suspension} \rightarrow 1 \text{ g amlodipine}$$

$$500 \text{ mL suspension} \rightarrow u$$

$$u = \frac{1 \text{ g amlodipine}}{200 \text{ mL suspension}} \times \frac{500 \text{ mL suspension}}{1}$$

$$= 2.5 \text{ g}$$

But the question is asking for the milligrams, so we convert the 2.5 g to milligrams. Thus,

$$1 \text{ g} \rightarrow 1{,}000 \text{ mg}$$

$$2.5 \text{ g} \rightarrow u$$

$$u = \frac{1{,}000 \text{ mg}}{1 \text{ g}} \times \frac{2.5 \text{ g}}{1}$$

$$= 2{,}500 \text{ mg}$$

Example 4.17

A pharmacist was ordered to prepare 1:400 solution of dextrose in distilled water. If the pharmacist only has 250 mg of dextrose, how many milliliters of the dextrose solution will the pharmacist be able to make?

Solution

The 1:400 ratio strength means that every 400 mL of the solution should contain 1 g of dextrose. This question is actually asking how many milliliters will contain 250 mg (or 0.25 g) of dextrose.

Using our proportion,

$$1 \text{ g dextrose} \rightarrow 400 \text{ mL solution}$$

$$250 \text{ mg dextrose} \rightarrow u$$

Realize that the units on the left are not the same and cannot be solved as is; therefore, the 250 mg must be converted to its gram equivalent.

Continuing

$$1{,}000 \text{ mg} \rightarrow 1 \text{ g}$$

$$250 \text{ mg} \rightarrow u$$

$$u = \frac{1\,g}{1{,}000\,mg} \times \frac{250\,mg}{1}$$

$$= 0.25 \text{ g}$$

250 mg is equivalent to 0.25 gram.

$$1 \text{ g dextrose} \rightarrow 400 \text{ mL solution}$$

$$0.25 \text{ g dextrose} \rightarrow u$$

$$u = \frac{400\,mL\,solution}{1\,g\,dextrose} \times \frac{0.25\,g\,dextrose}{1}$$

$$= 100 \text{ mL solution}$$

Example 4.18

The content of 2 capsules of amoxicillin (250 mg per capsule) was used to make 200 mL of amoxicillin suspension in simple syrup. What is the ratio strength of the resulting suspension?

Solution

The equivalence of 2 capsules of amoxicillin 250 mg is 2 × 250 mg = 500 mg amoxicillin. Therefore, the 200 mL of amoxicillin suspension contains the 500 mg amoxicillin. The question seeks to ask this: If 500 mg of amoxicillin is contained in 200 mL, how many milliliters of the suspension will contain just 1 g of amoxicillin? By mental math, the answer should be 400 mL.

Showing work

$$500 \text{ mg amoxicillin} \rightarrow 200 \text{ mL suspension}$$
$$1 \text{ g amoxicillin} \rightarrow u$$

The units on the left are not the same, so we convert 500 mg to its gram equivalent.

$$1,000 \text{ mg} \rightarrow 1 \text{ g}$$
$$500 \text{ mg} \rightarrow u$$

$$u = \frac{1\,g}{1,000\,mg} \times \frac{500\,mg}{1}$$

$$= 0.5 \text{ g amoxicillin}$$

$$0.5 \text{ g amoxicillin} \rightarrow 200 \text{ mL suspension}$$
$$1 \text{ g amoxicillin} \rightarrow u$$

$$u = \frac{200\,ml\,suspension}{0.5\,g\,amoxicillin} \times \frac{1\,g\,amoxicillin}{1}$$

$$= 400 \text{ mL suspension containing 1 g of the amoxicillin}$$

So ratio = 1:400.

Example 4.19

A certain solution is labeled 1:1,000. Convert the ratio strength to grams per milliliter.

Solution

This question is asking for the number of grams that will be present per milliliter of the solution. That is to say, if 1,000 mL of the formulation contains 1 g of the active ingredient, how many grams will be present in 1 mL of the suspension?

1,000 mL formulation → 1 g active ingredient (1:1000)

1 mL formulation → u

$$u = \frac{1 \text{ g active ingredient}}{1,000 \text{ mL formulation}} \times \frac{1 \text{ mL formulation}}{1}$$

= 0.001 g of active ingredient per mL of solution

Example 4.20

A properly reconstituted Keflex suspension in the pharmacy is labeled to contain 250 mg of cephalexin in every 5 mL of the suspension. Express this concentration as ratio strength.

Solution

First convert the 250 mg to its gram equivalent

$$1,000 \text{ mg} → 1 \text{ g}$$

$$250 \text{ mg} → u$$

$$u = \frac{1 \text{ g}}{1,000 \text{ mg}} \times \frac{250 \text{ mg}}{1}$$

= 0.25 gram

$$0.25 \text{ g} → 5 \text{ mL}$$

$$1 \text{ g} → u$$

$$u = \frac{5 \text{ mL}}{0.25 \text{ g}} \times \frac{1 \text{ g}}{1}$$

= 20 mL

Therefore, 20 mL of the suspension contains 1 g of the cephalexin. This defines the ratio strength.

Therefore, ratio strength is 1:20.

Freestyle/Fractional/Conventional Expression of Concentration

Concentration can also be expressed in its very simplified form: expressing the amount of active ingredient in any chosen unit per unit quantity of the formulation.

Azithromycin 125 mg/5 mL means that each 5 mL suspension contains 125 mg of azithromycin molecules.

This can be represented proportionally as

125 mg azithromycin → 5 mL suspension

or

5 mL suspension → 125 mg azithromycin

Using the proportions above, we can calculate the amount of azithromycin contained in any given volume of the suspension. We can also calculate the volume of the suspension that can contain any given amount of active ingredient (azithromycin).

Humalog insulin 100 units/mL means that each milliliter of the Humalog insulin suspension contains 100 units of the insulin.

100 units → 1 mL

or

1 mL → 100 units

Potassium chloride solution 20 mEq/5 mL means that each 5 mL of the solution contains 20 milliequivalents of potassium chloride.

20 mEq KCl → 5 mL

or

5 mL → 20 mEq KCl

We can use these proportions to calculate the amount of KCl in milliequivalents that will be contained in any given volume of the solution. We can also calculate the volume of the solutions that will contain any given milliequivalent of KCl.

Bisoprolol 5 mg/tab means that each tablet of the bisoprolol contains 5 mg of the active ingredient. Realize that each of the bisoprolol tablet weighs much more than 5 mg in the weighing scale because in addition to the active ingredient (bisoprolol), it contains other inactive ingredients (such as fillers, lubricants, disintegrants, bulking agents, etc.) Therefore, the 5 mg does not represent the total weight of the tablet but the amount of active ingredient in 1 tablet of the bisoprolol.

Hence, proportionally, we can say

5 mg bisoprolol active ingredient → 1 tab

1 tab → 5 mg bisoprolol active ingredient

Therefore, using the proportion, we can calculate the number of tablets that would contain a desired amount of the active ingredient. Using the lines of proportion above,also, we can calculate the amount of active ingredient if we know the number of tablets involved.

Example 4.21

Cephalexin suspension is labeled 250 mg/5 mL. If the physician wants the patient to receive 400 mg of cephalexin, how many milliliters should be given to the patient?

Solution

First, discover the relationship between the amount of medication (in milligrams) and the volume that contains it. Using proportion, we can say

250 mg cephalexin → 5 mL suspension

or

5 mL suspension → 250 mg cephalexin

The two expressions are exactly the same, but because we are looking for milliliters, we use the first one.

$$250 \text{ mg} \rightarrow 5 \text{ mL suspension}$$

$$400 \text{ mg} \rightarrow u$$

$$u = \frac{5 \text{ mL suspension}}{250 \text{ mg}} \times \frac{400 \text{ mg}}{1}$$

$$= 8 \text{ mL suspension}$$

A volume of 8 mL of cephalexin suspension 250 mg/5 mL will deliver 400 mg of cephalexin active ingredient.

Example 4.22

Dexamethasone injection is labeled dexamethasone 5 mg/8 mL. The physician instructed the nurse to administer 10 mL IM to a patient. How many milligrams of dexamethasone was the physician ordering to be administered to the patient?

Solution

Now our proportional relationship between the amount of dexamethasone and the volume of the solution containing it is

$$5 \text{ mg dexamethasone} \rightarrow 8 \text{ mL solution}$$

or

$$8 \text{ mL solution} \rightarrow 5 \text{ mg dexamethasone}$$

We are looking for milligrams, so we use the second expression.

$$8 \text{ mL solution} \rightarrow 5 \text{ mg dexamethasone}$$

$$10 \text{ mL solution} \rightarrow u$$

$$u = \frac{5 \text{ mg dexamethasone}}{8 \text{ mL solution}} \times \frac{10 \text{ mL solution}}{1}$$

$$= 6.25 \text{ mg dexamethasone}$$

Example 4.23

Levemir insulin has the label of 100 units/mL. The physician ordered that a patient should be injected with 30 units subcutaneously daily. How many milliliters should that be?

Solution

Since we are looking for the mL, our line of proportion goes like this:

$$100 \text{ units} \rightarrow 1 \text{ mL}$$

$$30 \text{ units} \rightarrow u$$

$$u = \frac{1\ mL}{100\ units} \times \frac{30\ units}{1}$$

$$= 0.3 \text{ mL}$$

Example 4.24

Carvedilol is available as 25 mg tablets. If the physician ordered 6.25 mg per dose, how many tablets should be given per dose?

Solution

We are looking for the number of tablets, so our line of proportion will have the tablets on the right-hand side.

$$25 \text{ mg} \rightarrow 1 \text{ tablet}$$

$$6.25 \text{ mg} \rightarrow u$$

$$u = \frac{1\ tablet}{25\ mg} \times \frac{6.25\ mg}{1}$$

$$= 0.25 \text{ tablet}$$

Example 4.25

The concentration of amlodipine suspension made by a pharmacist is 20 mg/mL. Convert this concentration to percentage strength.

Solution

Realize that percentage strength is defined as the amount of active ingredient (*in grams*) contained in 100 mL of the suspension. The question is therefore asking this: If 20 mg of medication is contained in 1 mL, how many grams will be contained in 100 mL of the suspension?

So we write our line of proportion:

$$20 \text{ mg} \rightarrow 1 \text{ mL}$$

or

$$1 \text{ mL} \rightarrow 20 \text{ mg}$$

Because we are looking for the amount (in milligrams) contained in 100 mL, we use the second line of proportion.

$$1 \text{ mL suspension} \rightarrow 20 \text{ mg amlodipine}$$
$$100 \text{ mL suspension} \rightarrow u$$

$$u = \frac{20 \text{ mg amlodipine}}{1 \text{ mL suspension}} \times \frac{100 \text{ mL suspension}}{1}$$

$$= 2{,}000 \text{ mg of amlodipine}$$

So 100 mL of suspension contains 2,000 mg of amlodipine. But percentage strength is defined by the amount of active ingredient (*in grams*) contained in 100 units of formulation. So the 2,000 mg must be converted to grams.

Thus,

$$1{,}000 \text{ mg} \rightarrow 1 \text{ gram}$$
$$2{,}000 \text{ mg} \rightarrow u$$

$$u = \frac{1 \, gram}{1,000 \, mg} \times \frac{2,000 \, mg}{1}$$

= 2 g contained in 100 mL of the suspension

Therefore, percentage strength is 2%.

Alternatively, we can convert the 20 mg to g initially and proceed with our calculations. Both ways, we will still arrive at the same answer.

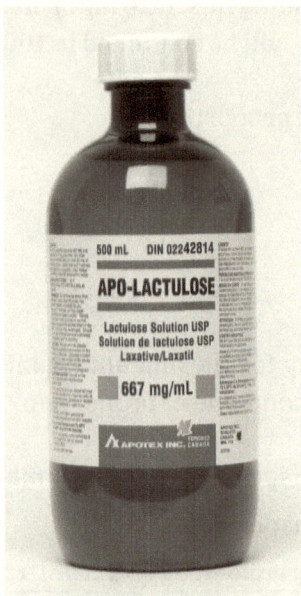

FIGURE 4.4 *Apo-Lactulose Solution USP:* Each mL of the formulation of the lactulose contains 667 mg of the active ingredient, lactulose. (Courtesy Apotex)

Example 4.26

Ranitidine pediatric liquid is labeled ranitidine 15 mg/mL. Convert this concentration to ratio strength.

Solution

Given that the ranitidine liquid contains 15 mg/mL, this question wants us to calculate how many milliliters of the suspension will contain just 1 g of ranitidine (active ingredient).

So, using our proportion,

$$15 \text{ mg ranitidine} \rightarrow 1 \text{ mL suspension}$$
$$1 \text{ g ranitidine} \rightarrow u$$

Realize that the units on the left are not the same, so one of them must be converted to the other to make a uniform unit.

Converting the 15 mg to grams (see chapter 2, "Interconversion of Units")

$$1{,}000 \text{ mg} \rightarrow 1 \text{ g}$$
$$15 \text{ mg} \rightarrow u$$

$$u = \frac{1\,g}{1{,}000\,mg} \times \frac{15\,mg}{1}$$

$$= 0.015 \text{ g}$$

The equivalent of 15 mg is 0.015 g.

Continuing

$$0.015 \text{ g ranitidine} \rightarrow 1 \text{ mL suspension}$$
$$1 \text{ g ranitidine} \rightarrow u$$

$$u = \frac{1\,mL \text{ suspension}}{0.015\,g\,ranitidine} \times \frac{1\,g\,ranitidine}{1}$$

$$= 66.667 \text{ mL suspension}$$

So 66.667 mL of the suspension contains 1 g of the active ingredient. Therefore, the ratio strength is 1:66.67.

Example 4.27

What amount of omeprazole will be used in making 2 pints of omeprazole suspension 2 mg / 5 mL?

Solution

First, we need to convert the pints to milliliters because the concentration is expressed in mg/mL.

$$1 \text{ pint} \rightarrow 480 \text{ mL}$$

$$2 \text{ pints} \rightarrow u$$

$$u = \frac{480 \, mL}{1 \, pint} \times \frac{2 \, pint}{1}$$

$$= 960 \text{ mL}$$

The question is actually asking this: If 2 mg omeprazole is contained in 5 mL, how many milligrams will be contained in 960 mL?

Using our proportion,

$$5 \text{ mL} \rightarrow 2 \text{ mg (keeping mg to the right)}$$

$$960 \text{ mL} \rightarrow u$$

$$u = \frac{2 \, mg}{5 \, mL} \times \frac{960 \, mL}{1}$$

$$= 384 \text{ mg omeprazole}$$

Example 4.28

A physician authorized 2 tablespoonfuls of amoxicillin suspension labeled amoxicillin 125 mg / 5 mL to be given to a child as a single dose. How many milligrams will the child receive from the single dose of 2 tablespoonfuls?

Solution

First, the 2 tablespoonfuls need to be converted to milliliters because the strength of the suspension is in mg/mL.

$$1 \text{ tbsp} \rightarrow 15 \text{ mL}$$
$$2 \text{ tbsp} \rightarrow 30 \text{ mL}$$

Hence, the question is asking, if 5 mL of the suspension contains 125 mg, how many milligrams will be contained in 30 mL (2 tablespoonfuls)?

So again, using our proportion,

$$5 \text{ mL suspension} \rightarrow 125 \text{ mg amoxicillin}$$
$$30 \text{ mL suspension} \rightarrow u$$
$$u = \frac{125 \; mg \; amoxicillin}{5 \; mL \; suspension} \times \frac{30 \; mL \; suspension}{1}$$
$$= 750 \text{ mg of amoxicillin}$$

An amount of 2 tablespoonfuls of the suspension will supply 750 mg of the medication.

Example 4.29

You receive the following order:

Rx

Metformin tablets 500 mg

Sig: 2 tablets once daily for 10 days.

(Metformin is available in the pharmacy as 500 mg tablets.)

How many grams total will be dispensed to the patient for 10 days?

Solution

First, calculate the number of tablets authorized to be dispensed to the patient.

$$\text{Number of tablets} = 2 \text{ tablets} \times 10$$
$$= 20 \text{ tablets}$$

Each tablet contains 500 mg of metformin, so our proportion goes

$$1 \text{ tablet} \rightarrow 500 \text{ mg}$$
$$20 \text{ tablets} \rightarrow u$$
$$u = \frac{500\ mg}{1\ tablet} \times \frac{20\ tablets}{1}$$
$$= 10,000 \text{ mg}$$

This amount is then converted to grams.

$$1,000 \text{ mg} \rightarrow 1 \text{ g}$$
$$10,000 \text{ mg} \rightarrow u$$
$$u = \frac{1\,g}{1,000\ mg} \times \frac{10,000\ mg}{1}$$
$$= 10 \text{ g}$$

Example 4.30

An intravenous infusion contains 50% dextrose in distilled water. How many milliliters of the infusion should be administered to provide a patient with 200 g of dextrose?

Solution

A 50% dextrose solution means that every 100 mL of the dextrose solution contains 50 g of dextrose. This question is then asking for the volume of the solution that will contain 200 g of the dextrose.

Using our proportion,

$$50 \text{ g dextrose} \rightarrow 100 \text{ mL solution}$$

$$200 \text{ g dextrose} \rightarrow u$$

$$u = \frac{100 \text{ mL solution}}{50 \text{ g dextrose}} \times \frac{200 \text{ g dextrose}}{1}$$

$$= 400 \text{ mL solution}$$

400 mL of the solution will deliver 200 g of the dextrose.

Chapter 4 Practice Questions

1. A pharmacist made 500 mL 7% suspension of metoclopramide. How many milligrams of metoclopramide powder was used in the preparation?

2. Express 1:500 solution of sodium bicarbonate as percentage strength.

3. A physician ordered 1:1,000 solution of Zofran with instructions to administer 8 mg once daily. How many milliliters should be administered to the patient once daily?

4. Contained in 10 g of a topical formulation is 500 mg of minoxidil powder. What is the percentage strength of the formulation? (Active ingredient is minoxidil)

5. A physician orders 375 mg of cephalexin three times daily for 10 days for a child with a skin infection. If the drug is available as cephalexin 125 mg / 5 mL, how many teaspoons should be given to the child per day?

6. A physician orders 1,000 mcg vitamin B_{12} injection for a patient per month. If B_{12} injection is available as 1 mg/mL, calculate how many milliliters should be administered to the patient per month.

7. If you have a 12% solution of potassium chloride, how many milligrams of potassium chloride will be present in 1 mL of the solution?

8. Sodium bicarbonate solution is labeled with percentage strength of 8.4%. How many milligrams of the medication is contained in every milliliter of the solution?

9. If a drug is labeled 20 mg / 6 mL, how many grams of the drug powder should be used in making 600 mL of the suspension?

10. A pharmacist prepared 10 ounces of amlodipine suspension labeled 15 mg / 8 mL. How many grams of amlodipine powder did he use in the preparation?

11. Ranitidine suspension comes as 20 mg/mL. Convert this concentration to ratio strength.

12. A pharmacist dissolved 900 mg of a drug powder in enough distilled water to make 1 pint of solution. Calculate the percentage strength.

13. Morphine sulfate injection contains 10 mg of morphine in every 1 mL of the solution. Express this concentration as ratio strength.

14. You were required to make 300 g of 40% salicylic acid in Vaseline. You look at the shelf only to discover that you have only one full bottle of 5 g salicylic powder. What is the maximum quantity of the salicylic acid you can make?

15. A physician prescribed 6.25 mg of carvedilol. Carvedilol is available as tablets, each containing 25 mg carvedilol. How many tablets of the 25 mg should be administered?

16. A physician ordered 1:100 solution of KCl with instructions to administer 10 mg of the active ingredient to the patient. How many milliliters should be administered?

17. A cream contains 6 g of menthol made up to 60 g with a topical cream base. What is the percent concentration?

18. How many milligrams of aluminum acetate is required to prepare 500 mL of 1:2,000 solution?

19. If you are requested to prepare 1:400 sodium chloride solution, how many milliliters will you be able to prepare with 500 mg of NaCl crystals?

20. Insulin regular comes as 100 units/mL. If the physician wanted the patient to self-inject 0.15 mL, how many units should that be?

21. A physician ordered 10 mL of ranitidine 2% suspension to be administered to a child. How many milligrams of ranitidine is contained in the administered volume?

22. How many milliliters of 1:50 solution of epinephrine will deliver 50 mg of the active ingredient (adrenaline)?

23. A pharmaceutical solution contains solid dissolved in distilled water. The ratio strength is 1:2,000. What amount of the solid in milligrams will be contained in every 1 mL of the solution?

24. If 50 mg of a certain drug is contained in 5 mL of the formulation, calculate the percentage strength of the formulation.

25. How many grams of diclofenac powder will be needed to make 80 g of 10% diclofenac gel?

26. A pharmacist wants to add 50 mg of adrenaline into 500 mL 50% dextrose water. Unfortunately, adrenaline is not available as a pure powder but is only available as a stock solution labeled 12 mg / 5 mL. How many milliliters of this stock solution must be put into the dextrose water?

27. You were given a preparation that contains 1,500 mg of mannitol dissolved in water to produce 150 mL. Express the concentration as percentage strength.

28. An amount of 500 mg dextrose powder was mixed in enough distilled water to make 200 mL. What is the ratio strength of the solution?

29. During a laboratory experiment, 2 students were told to share 500 mL of 20 mg/mL solution at the ratio of 3:2. How many milligrams will be contained in each student's share of the solutions?

30. To make 40 mL of solution, 8 g of an active drug powder is dissolved in sterile water. What is the percentage concentration of the resulting solution?

31. A certain anabolic steroid contains 200 mg of medication in every 5 mL of the solution. Convert this concentration to ratio strength.

32. A pharmacist added 100 mL of distilled water to 400 mL of 1:1,000 solution of NaCl. What is the new ratio strength formed by that dilution?

33. A prefilled syringe of a liquid medication is labeled 27 mg/6 mL. If the volume of the liquid is 3 teaspoons, how many milligrams of the medication is contained in the prefilled syringe?

34. A physician orders 20 mg of a drug. If the drug is available as 5 mg/8 mL, how many milliliters should be dispensed?

35. An intravenous infusion is labeled 5% dextrose in distilled water. How many liters of the infusion should be administered if the physician requests that patient should receive only 0.55 pounds of the dextrose?

36. If you mixed 15 g of clindamycin powder with 165 g of a neutral base such as Diffusimax, what is the percentage concentration of the resultant clindamycin gel?

37. How many milligrams of ammonium chloride is contained in 300 mL of 1:10,000 of ammonia chloride solution?

38. If the labeled strength of a suspension is 150 mg / 8 mL, how many milligrams of the drug will be contained in 1 gallon of the suspension?

39. What volume of Cefzil 125 mg / 5 mL will yield 5 g of the active ingredient (cefprozil)?

40. Blended with 5 g of solid powdered medicinal ingredient is 195 g of a base. Calculate the ratio strength of the resulting topical preparation.

41. You receive the following prescription:

    Rx

    Fucidin cream 2%

    Apply approximately 2 g to affected area as needed.

    Approximately what amount of the active ingredient
    is delivered to the skin per application?

42. What is the gram amount of potassium permanganate in 300 mL
    of a 1:50 solution of potassium permanganate?

43. The dosage of a medication requires that the patient should take
    3 mL of the medication containing 280 mg / 8 mL. How many
    milligrams does the patient receive per dose?

44. A pharmacist prepared a 5% menthol cream. Convert this
    concentration to ratio strength.

45. A pharmacist prepared 300 mL of amlodipine suspension
    5 mg/3 mL. He accidentally spilled 1 tablespoonful of the
    suspension. How many milligrams were lost as a result of the spill?

46. A compounded amlodipine oral pediatric liquid is labeled 0.1%.
    If a child is to receive 2 teaspoonfuls, how many milligrams will
    the child receive?

47. A powdered medicinal ingredient was mixed with a topical base
    to make a cream of ratio strength 1:50. What is the percentage
    strength of the topical cream formed?

48. When reconstituted, azithromycin suspension is labeled 200 mg/5 mL. Convert this concentration to ratio strength.

49. A pharmacy assistant prepared a 7.5% solution of potassium permanganate. How many grams of potassium permanganate will be contained in 3 cups of the solution?

50. A certain anabolic steroid solution comes as 1,000 mg / 5 mL. If the physician wants the patient to inject 0.4 g of the medication, how many milliliters should the patient inject?

★ Star Question ★

You have 3 different bottles of dexamethasone suspension made with the same vehicle as follows:

Bottle A is 165 mL of 5 mg / 3 mL suspension

Bottle B is 200 mL of 1:2,000 ratio strength suspension

Bottle C is 235 mL of a 2.5% suspension

The contents of these bottles are mixed together in a bowl. How many milliliters of this mixture should be given to a child as a single dose if the child is to receive 62.5 mg of dexamethasone as a single dose?

Answers to Chapter 4
Practice Questions

1. 35,000 mg metoclopramide
2. 0.2%
3. 8 mL
4. 5%
5. 9 tsp
6. 1 mL
7. 120 mg
8. 84 mg
9. 2 g
10. 0.5625 g
11. 1:50
12. 0.1875%
13. 1:100
14. 12.5 g
15. ¼ tab
16. 1 mL
17. 10%
18. 250 mg
19. 200 mL
20. 15 units
21. 200 mg
22. 2.5 mL
23. 0.5 mg
24. 1%
25. 8 g
26. 20.83 mL
27. 1%
28. 1:400
29. 3:2 = 6,000 mg:4,000 mg
30. 20%
31. 1:25
32. 1:1,250

33. 67.5 mg
34. 32 mL
35. 5 L
36. 8.33%
37. 30 mg
38. 72,000 mg
39. 200 mL
40. 1:40
41. 0.04 g (40 mg)
42. 6 g
43. 105 mg
44. 1:20
45. 25 mg
46. 10 mg
47. 2%
48. 1:25
49. 54 g
50. 2 mL

Solution to Star Question

First, we need to get the total volume contributed by the 3 bottles of suspension.

$$= 165 \text{ mL} + 200 \text{ mL} + 235 \text{ mL}$$

$$= 600 \text{ mL total volume when the contents of the 3 bottles are mixed together}$$

Next, we need to get the total amount of dexamethasone contributed by the 3 bottles of suspension:

Dexamethasone in A + Dexamethasone in B + Dexamethasone in C

Dexamethasone in Bottle A (165 mL of 5 mg / 3 mL suspension)

$$3 \text{ mL suspension} \rightarrow 5 \text{ mg dexamethasone}$$
$$165 \text{ mL suspension} \rightarrow u$$

$$u = \frac{5 \ mg \ dexamethasone}{3 \ mL \ suspension} \times \frac{165 \ mL \ suspension}{1}$$

$$= 275 \ mg \ Dexamethasone$$

Dexamethasone in Bottle B (200 mL of 1:2,000 ratio strength suspension)

2,000 mL suspension → 1 g dexamethasone

200 mL suspension → u

$$u = \frac{1 \ g \ dexamethasone}{2,000 \ mL \ suspension} \times \frac{200 \ mL \ suspension}{1}$$

$$= 0.1 \ g$$

$$= 100 \ mg$$

Dexamethasone in Bottle C (235 mL of a 2.5% suspension)

100 mL suspension → 2.5 g dexamethasone

235 mL suspension → u

$$u = \frac{2.5 \ g \ dexamethasone}{100 \ mL \ suspension} \times \frac{235 \ mL \ suspension}{1}$$

$$= 5.875 \ g$$

$$= 5,875 \ mg$$

Total amount of dexamethasone is

275 mg + 100 mg + 5,875 mg

= 6,250 mg of dexamethasone all inside the
600 mL of the mixed suspension

So we can say that 6,250 mg of dexamethasone is contained inside 600 mL of the suspension mixed.

If a child is to receive 62.5 mg, what volume of the mix should be given?

6,250 mg dexamethasone → 600 mL suspension

62.5 mg dexamethasone → u

$$u = \frac{600 \ mL \ suspension}{6,250 \ mg \ dexamethasone} \times \frac{62.5 \ mg \ dexamethasone}{1}$$

= 6 mL of the suspension mix

CHAPTER 5

Interpretation of Medication Orders and Prescriptions

Objectives

At the end of this chapter, students should be able to do the following:

- Demonstrate understanding of the etymologies of some expressions used in prescription writing
- Transcribe prescriptions written by competent professionals
- Determine dosages in a prescription after prescription interpretation

The ability to understand and interpret a prescription is one of the essential skills of any professional (the pharmacist, pharmacy technician or pharmacy assistant, nurse, etc.) who wishes to work with medications and prescriptions.

A prescription is an authorization issued by a physician or other qualified prescriber to the pharmacist to dispense the desired medication to a patient. It is an order that is called in (verbal), written, or faxed for a specific patient by a medical professional who has authority to prescribe.

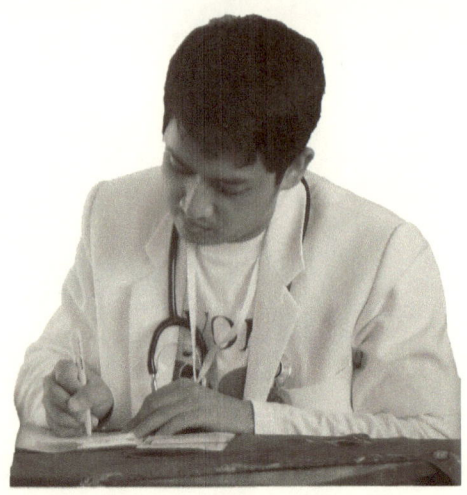

FIGURE 5.1 *A Physician Writing a Prescription:* Although prescriptions should be written in English language, use of Latinized expressions in prescriptions is still common. It is therefore the duty of a medical professional (example, pharmacist) to interpret the signature (sig) of a prescription into a language that is comprehensible to the patient.

There are certain requirements that complete a prescription, and every pharmacy team member should be aware of these for the safety of the public.

Every prescription must have the following parts:

- The prescriber's information
- The patient's information
- The medication information
- The date
- The prescriber's signature (if prescription is not verbal)

The contemporary pharmacy practice has its roots from the apothecaries. Historically, the apothecaries were those who formulated and dispensed medications to doctors and patients in the medieval age.

The language of the apothecaries had its roots in Latin, which was connected to the defunct Roman Empire. The modern-day medical practice is an inheritance from the apothecaries. Thus, the use of Latin in the writing of prescriptions has been inherited by the contemporary medical practice.

Although prescriptions in Canada and other North American countries should be written in the English language, use of expressions from Latin roots is still common. This style of writing literally compresses and abridges the prescription information and, at the same time, somewhat makes the prescription language esoteric.

Therefore, any health professional wishing to work in the medical field (doctors, pharmacists, assistants, and technicians) must be conversant with these expressions. This is because the skill is needed for writing, interpreting, and translating the expressions into a language that is comprehensible to the patients in a way that eliminates errors and ensures that the right patient gets the right medication, right dosage and through the right route of administration.

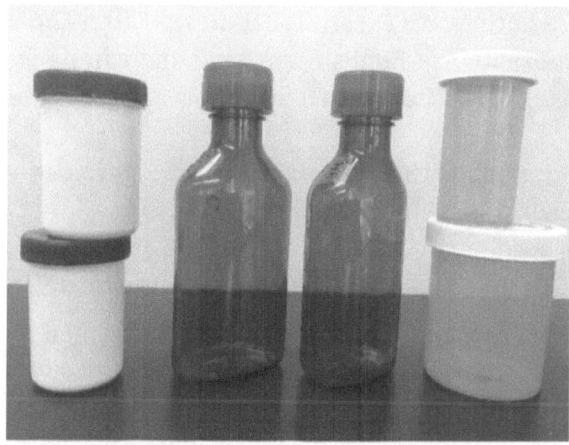

FIGURE 5.2 *Containers for Dispensing Medications:* After the interpretation of a prescription, during the packaging, the professional should be able to determine the most appropriate container in which the medication should be dispensed. Left - Ointment jars used for dispensing creams, ointment, pastes and other topical preparations. Middle - calibrated amber colored plastic containers for dispensing liquid oral preparations like suspensions, solutions and elixirs. Right - Containers for dispensing solid oral formulations like tablets or capsules. The regulation requires these containers to have a child safety cap unless the patient expressly requests non-safety containers with a written consent.

Latinized Expressions

In this book, efforts have been made to arrange the Latinized expressions in certain groups that will make it easy for the readers' understanding of the expressions. Efforts have also been made to include the literal interpretation of some of the Latinized expression as well as trace the contemporary English words/expressions that have their roots in such Latinized words/expressions.

Ante. This is a Latin prefixal form of preposition and adverb, which means "before." It has become part of the English language. It is seen in words like *antenatal* ("before birth") and *anteceded* ("to go before").

Cibos. Cibos is a Latin noun meaning "food." It has become part of the English language, seen in words like *cibophobia* ("fear of food") and *ciborium* ("a vessel for holding Eucharistic bread").

Post. This is a Latin word (prefix) that means "after" or "later." It has been imported into the English language and can be found in such words as *postnatal* ("after birth") and *postwar* ("after the war").

These would explain the meaning of some Latinized expressions found in prescriptions like

AC (ante cibum), which means "before food," and

PC (post cibum), which means "after food."

Auris. In Latin, the ear is called Auris. The English language has borrowed this Latin expression in everyday usage, with terms such as *auricular* ("related to the ear or sense of hearing").

Dexter. This is a Latin noun meaning "on the right." English language has borrowed *dexter* in its everyday use, with modification to *'dextral'* ("of or relating to the right"). The sugar *dextrose* is so named because the molecule has the property of rotating the plain of a polarized light ray to the right.

Sinistra. This Latin noun means "left." Because left is the opposite of right and is associated with wrong, bad, or somewhat evil, the English language has borrowed *sinistra* (with some modification of the word to 'sinister') for everyday use to mean "on the left," "unlucky," "evil," or "capable of causing harm." An example would be the phrase *"sinister forces"* (evil forces).

These would explain the interpretation of the following Latinized expressions related to the ear, which are used in prescriptions:

AD (Auris dexter) — right ear

AS (Auris sinistra) — left ear

Meridies. This is a Latin word that means "noon." The English language modified this word to *meridian*, which means midday. *Ante meridiem* therefore literally means "before noon" and is considered to mean "morning," and *post meridiem* is considered to mean "evening."

This explains the meaning of the following Latinized expressions:

AM (ante meridiem) — morning

PM (post meridiem) — evening

Aqua. This means "water" in Latin. The adjective form of the word, *aquatic*, is an English word imported from Latin and means "from or related to water."

Bis. This is a Latin prefix or suffix describing the second instance of a thing or simply meaning "twice." English has inherited this word to also mean "twice." It is used in music as a direction to repeat. Furthermore, it was modified in English as prefix *bi-* to suggest double—*bilingual* ("two languages"), *bilateral, bifocal.*

Die. This is a Latin noun that means "day" (the twenty-four-hour day). Therefore, Latin expression *bis in die* literally means "twice in a day" and is commonly translated in prescription as twice daily. It is used to mean "two" when naming some organic compounds.

BID (bis in die) — twice daily

Cum. This is a Latin word used as a preposition or conjunction that mostly means "with." This Latin word has been inherited by the English language to mean "plus" or "along with." It is usually used as a hyphenated phrase. "Mr. Anderson is a doctor-cum-writer" means the same thing as "Mr. Anderson is a doctor as well as a writer."

CC (cum cibum) — with food

Fiat. In Latin, this word means "let it be done." In the English language, *fiat* has been borrowed from Latin and means "a binding edict issued by a person in command."

Ft (fiat) — let it be made

Example

Diclo 10%

Ft 200 grams (make 200 grams of diclo 10%)

Gutta. This is written as *gtt* in prescription and is a Latin word for "drop." The English word *gutter* ("a channel made for carrying raindrops away") probably took its root from this Latin word *gutta*.

ii *gtt* — 2 drops

Hora. This is a Latin word that means "hour" in the English language. The word *hour* in the English language has its roots in Latin and old French.

Somni. This is a Latin word that means "sleep" in the English language. The English language has borrowed the root word *somni* in its everyday use in words related to sleep such as *somnolent* ("likely to induce sleep") and *somnolence* ("the quality or state of being drowsy"). Therefore, *hora somni (HS)* means literally "hour of sleep," and in pharmacy, it is interpreted as bedtime.

HS (hora somni) — hour of sleep / bedtime

Nocte. *Nocte* is a Latin word that means "night." In English, this word has been borrowed and used in words having to do with night. E.g., *nocturnal* animals are animals that are active at night but relatively inactive during the day.

Nocte — at night

Oculus. This is a Latin word that means "eye." The English language has borrowed this as a root word in expressions related to the eye. *Oculist* is an English word meaning "optometrist."

OD (oculus dextra) — right eye

OS (oculus sinistra) — left eye

OU (oculus uterque) — both eyes (each eye)

Uterque — a Latin word that means "both"

Per. This is a Latin word that means "by" or "through." We encounter *per* in the English language to denote "through" or "by means of." *Per annum* means "through one year."

Os. This is a Latin word that means "mouth." The English language has borrowed this word in anatomy to denote "the opening of the cervix" (literally "mouth of the cervix"). The anatomical tube connecting the mouth and the stomach (called oesophagus) probably got its name from this root.

PO (per OS) — by mouth

Pro re nata (PRN). This is a Latin expression that is literally interpreted as meaning "when the circumstances arise." It is written as *PRN* in prescriptions and is interpreted as "when needed" or "as needed."

PRN (pro re nata) – As needed.

Quaque. This is a Latin expression that means "every." *Quaque* is written in prescription as the letter *q*, hence

QAM (quaque ante meridien) — every morning

QPM (quaque post meridien) — every evening

QH (quaque hora) — every hour

QHS (quaque hora somni) — every night at bedtime

Q1H (quaque 1 hora) — every 1 hour

QD (quaque die) — everyday

Statim. This is expressed as *stat* in prescriptions, which means "at once."

Stat (statim) — at once or immediately

Ter. This is a Latin expression meaning "thrice." English has modified this to the prefix *tri-*, used in words like *tricycle*, *triune*, and *tripod*.

TID (ter in die) — thrice in a day or three times daily

The explanations of these latinized expressions are not in any way exhaustive. They are, however, limited to what is needed in this book as far as prescription writing is concerned.

Expressions Related to the Route of Administration

IM — intramuscular

SC, SQ — subcutaneously

IV — intravenously

ID — intradermal

IN — intranasal (nose)

PV — per vagina (vaginally)

PR — per rectum (rectally)

Bucc — buccally (inside the cheek)

Top — topical

PO — by mouth

SL — sublingually

NPO — nothing by mouth

Expressions Related to Frequency

q week — every week

q month — every month

qh — every hour

q2h — every 2 hours

q4h — every 4 hours

q6h — every 6 hours

q8h — every 8 hours

Expressions Related to Number of Times a Day

OD — once daily

QD — daily

BID — twice a day

TID — three times a day

QID — four times a day

EOD, QOD — every other day

PRN — as needed, when required

AM — morning

PM — evening

QAM — every morning

QPM — every evening

QHS — every day at bedtime

Q4H — every 4 hours

QWK – every week

Expressions Related to Specific Times

CC — with food (*cc* also means ml)

AC — before meal

PC — after meals

HS — hour of sleep *or* bedtime

Stat — at once, immediately

Expressions Related to Form of Administration / Dosage Forms

Tab — tablet

Cap — capsules

Gtt — drops

Liq — liquid

Syr — syrup

Elix — elixir

Ung — ointment

Supp — suppository

Inj — injectable

Crm — cream

Lot — lotion

Nebul — spray

Pulv — powder

Susp — suspension

Expressions Related to the Measurement of Medication

mg — milligram

mL — milliliter

g, gm — gram

k, kg — kilogram

mcg — microgram

tsp — teaspoon

c — cup

lb — pound

in (") — inch

ft (') — foot

oz — ounce

pt — pint

qt — quart

mEq — milliequivalent

u — unit

gr — grain

tbsp — tablespoon

tsp — teaspoon

Expressions Related to the Eye (Eye = *Oculus* in Latin)

OD (Oculus dexter) — right eye

OS (Oculus sinistra) — left eye

OU (Oculus uterque) — both eyes

Expressions Related to the Ear (Ear = Auris in Latin)

AD (Auris dexter) — right ear

AS (Auris sinistra) — left ear

AU (Auris uterque) — both ears

Other General Abbreviations

$\bar{c}$ — with

$\bar{s}$ — without

= — equal

≠ — not equal

< — less than

> — greater than

Rx — prescription, take this drug

OTC — over the counter

VO — verbal order

TO — telephone order

NKA — no known allergy

NKDA — no known drug allergy

UD — as directed

$\overline{aa}$ — of each

↑ — increase

↓ — decrease

Non Rep — do not repeat

Noct, Nocte — by night

AAA — apply to affected area

Amt — amount

Aq — water

Comp — compound

Ft — make, let it be made

Hr — hour

IU — international unit

MDU — to be used as directed

Mitte — send

Per — by or through

qs — quantity sufficient

Rep — repeat

Sig — write on label

SOB — shortness of breath

SS — one half

X — times

Amp — ampoule

I — one

II — two

III — three

IV — four

V — five

Etc.

$\dfrac{X}{7}$, X = number of days

$\dfrac{X}{52}$, X = number of weeks

$\dfrac{X}{12}$, X = number of months

Chapter 5 Practice Examples

Interpret the following prescriptions.

Example 5.1

> Cap.amoxicillin 500 mg
> Sig: ii tid uf
>> M: 60 No Rep

Interpretation

Capsule amoxicillin 500 mg

Take 2 capsules three times daily until finished.

Send 60 capsules with no repeat.

Example 5.2

> Tab naproxen EC 500 mg
> Sig: ii BID PC
>> M: 60 tablets

Interpretation

Tab naproxen enteric coated 500 mg.

Take 2 tablets twice daily after meals.

Give 60 tablets.

Example 5.3

> Gtt Ciprodex otic
> Sig: iv gtt AD QID UD
> > M: 7.5 mL

Interpretation

Ciprodex eardrops

Instill 4 drops into the right ear four times daily as directed.

Give 7.5 mL.

Example 5.4

> Gtt Tobradex ophth
> Sig: 1 gtt OU TID $\dfrac{10}{7}$

Interpretation

Tobradex eye drops

Instill 1 drop into both eyes three times daily for ten days

Example 5.5

> Tab Synthroid 100 mcg
> Sig: i po QAM ½ Hour AC
>
> $$\dfrac{3}{52}$$

Interpretation

Synthroid tablet 100 microgram

Take one tablet by mouth daily in the morning ½ hour before meals for 3 weeks.

Example 5.6

> Ellix Cotridin cough
>
> Sig: 10 mL po cc QHS PRN
>
> $$\frac{1}{12}$$

Interpretation

Cotridin elixir for cough

Take 10 mL orally at bedtime with meal as needed

Supply for 1 month.

Example 5.7

> Compound diclofenac 10% in PLO gel
>
> Sig: AAA TID right knee PRN
>
> Ft: 100 grams

Interpretation

Make 10% diclofenac in PLO gel.

Apply to the affected area of the right knee three times daily as needed.

Make 100 grams.

Example 5.8

> Inj Zostavax
>
> Sig: 0.65 mL SC stat
>
> M: 1 bottle

Interpretation

Zostavax injection

Inject 0.65 mL subcutaneously at once.

Supply 1 bottle.

Example 5.9

> Tab Imovane 7.5 mg
> Sig: ss po HS PRN
>
> $\dfrac{3}{12}$ rep ×4

Interpretation

Imovane tablet

Take $\dfrac{1}{2}$ tablets by mouth at bedtime as needed.

Supply for 3 months with four repeats.

Example 5.10

> Ung Betaderm 0.1%
> Sig: AAA sparingly TID eczema lesions
>   M: 30 g Rep ×2

Interpretation

Betaderm ointment 0.1%

Apply to affected area sparingly three times a day to eczematous lesions.

Supply 30 g with 2 repeats.

Example 5.11

> Tab Ativan SL 1 mg
> Sig: 2 SL stat 1 hr prior to dental appt UD
>> M 2 tablets ×3 repeats

Interpretation

Sublingual Ativan tablets 1 mg.

Dissolve 2 tablets at once under the tongue one hour prior to dental appointment as directed.

Supply 2 tablets with 3 repeats.

Example 5.12

> Crm Canesten
> Sig: App top. UD PRN
>> M: 50 g

Interpretation

Canesten cream

Apply topically as directed as needed.

Supply 50 grams.

Example 5.13

> Tab Vagifem 10 mcg
> Sig: i ins pv 3 × Qweek UD
>> $$\frac{3}{12}$$

Interpretation

Vagifem vaginal tablet 10 mcg

Insert 1 tablet vaginally 3 times per week as directed.

Supply for 3 months.

Example 5.14

> Anusol sup
> Sig: ins 1 PR QHS UD
>   12

Interpretation

Anusol suppository

Insert 1 suppository rectally nightly at bedtime as directed.

Give 12.

Example 5.15

> Tab Tylenol #3
> Sig: i–ii po Q4-6H PRNP
> $\dfrac{10}{7}$

Interpretation

Tylenol number 3

Take one or two tablets by mouth every 4 to 6 hours as needed for pain for 10 days.

Example 5.16

> Nystatin oral susp. 100,000 units/mL
> Sig: Agit then swish and swallow 5 mL
> Q3-4H UF
>> M: 50 mL

Interpretation

Nystatin oral suspension 100,000 units/mL

Shake well and then swish and swallow 5 mL every 3 to 4 hours until finished.

Give 50 mL.

Example 5.17

> Azithromycin (Z-pack) 250 mg
> Sig: 500 mg po stat, then 250 mg QD
> Days 2 to 4
>> M: 6 tabs

Interpretation

Azithromycin 250 mg tablets

Take 2 tablets orally at once on day 1, then take one tablet orally once daily for days 2 to 4.

Give 6 tablets.

Example 5.18

> Bisoprolol 5 mg
>
> Sig: ss po BID UD
>
> Not to take if BP $< \dfrac{110}{70}$ or pulse ≤ 60
>
> M: 30

Interpretation:

Bisoprolol tablets 5 mg.

Take $\dfrac{1}{2}$ tablet orally twice daily as directed.

Do not take if blood pressure is less than $\dfrac{110}{70}$ or pulse less than or equal to 60.

Give 30 tablets.

Chapter 5 Practice Questions

For the following real-time community handwritten prescriptions, interpret the sig and write down inside a bracket the possible Indication(s) of the medications prescribed.

①

Patient Name:_____

Patient Address:_____

Date:___Today_____

Age:_____

℞

Tab Bisoprolol 5mg

Sig: ss̄ PO QD if HR ↑ UD

#50 tabs.

Refill: ∅

②

DR. JOE KINGSON, M.D, F.R.C.P
Jophil Medical Clinic
Fountain Plaza, 54 Broadstreet SW,
Calgary, AB. T3X OP3
Phone: 587 724 1193

Patient Name:_____ Date: Today_____

Patient Address:_____ Age:_____

R_x

Amoxil 8 p.
250 mg TID X
10 days.

Refill: ∅

③

Hahneman Family Clinic
Dr. C.C. Egbus, M.D
158 95th Avenue Bearspaw Ranchlands
Northwest Calgary, AB. T0Y 5N7
Phone: 403 103 2359

Patient Name:_____ Date: Today_____

Patient Address:_____ Age:_____

R_x

Tab Imovane 7.5mg
ss PO QAM, 1 po HS PRN
M: 300 tablets

Refill: 2

④

DR. JOE KINGSON, M.D, F.R.C.P
Jophil Medical Clinic
Fountain Plaza, 54 Broadstreet SW,
Calgary, AB. T3X OP3
Phone: 587 724 1193

Patient Name:_____ Date:___Today_____

Patient Address:_____ Age:_____

R_x

Tab biaxin XL 500mg
Sig: ii PO OD UF
#20

Refill:___∅___

⑤

Hahneman Family Clinic
Dr. C.C. Egbus, M.D
158 95th Avenue Bearspaw Ranchlands
Northwest Calgary, AB. T0Y 5N7
Phone: 403 103 2359

Patient Name:_____ Date:___Today_____

Patient Address:_____ Age:___70yrs_____

R_x

Cap Advil 400mg Liquogel
Sig: T PO Q4-6H Prnp
#100 Capsules

Refill:___∅___

⑥

DR. JOE KINGSON, M.D, F.R.C.P

Jophil Medical Clinic

Fountain Plaza, 54 Broadstreet SW,
Calgary, AB. T3X OP3
Phone: 587 724 1193

Patient Name:_____ Date:___Today___
Patient Address:_____ Age:_____

℞

TAB ANAPROX DS 550MG
SIG: ṫ PO BID CC PRN
M: 90 TABS

Refill: 2

⑦

Hahneman Family Clinic

Dr. C.C. Egbus, M.D

158 95th Avenue Bearspaw Ranchlands
Northwest Calgary, AB. T0Y 5N7
Phone: 403 103 2359

Patient Name:_____ Date:___TODAY___
Patient Address:_____ Age:_____

℞

1y Zostavax
Sig: 0.65ml SC stat UD
M: One dose

Refill: Ø

⑧

DR. JOE KINGSON, M.D, F.R.C.P
Jophil Medical Clinic
Fountain Plaza, 54 Broadstreet SW,
Calgary, AB. T3X OP3
Phone: 587 724 1193

Patient Name:_____

Patient Address:_____

Date: Today

Age:_____

R_x

Tab Colchicine 0.6 mg

Sig: ꞏ̇꞉̇ī̇ PO Q2-4H PC Prnp Cont

#30

Refill: Ø

Hahneman Family Clinic
Dr. C.C. Egbus, M.D
158 95th Avenue Bearspaw Ranchlands
Northwest Calgary, AB. T0Y 5N7
Phone: 403 103 2359

⑨

Patient Name:_____

Patient Address:_____

Date: Today

Age:_____

R_x

① Tramacet - ῑ ꞉̇ῑῑ tabs PO

Q 4-6h PRN

mitte: 50 tabs

Refill: 2

⑩

DR. JOE KINGSON, M.D, F.R.C.P
Jophil Medical Clinic
Fountain Plaza, 54 Broadstreet SW,
Calgary, AB. T3X OP3
Phone: 587 724 1193

Patient Name:_____   Date:___Today___
Patient Address:_____   Age:_____

R_x

Ung. Erythromycin ophth.
Sig: App 1 strip OS lower eye lids BID
M: 3.5 grams

Refill:_____

Hahneman Family Clinic
Dr. C.C. Egbus, M.D
158 95th Avenue Bearspaw Ranchlands
Northwest Calgary, AB. T0Y 5N7
Phone: 403 103 2359

⑪

Patient Name:_____   Date:___Today___
Patient Address:_____   Age:_____

R_x

Annual Suppository
Ins 1 PR Nocte uD
#24

Refill: Ø

DR. JOE KINGSON, M.D, F.R.C.P
Jophil Medical Clinic
Fountain Plaza, 54 Broadstreet SW,
Calgary, AB. T3X OP3
Phone: 587 724 1193

Patient Name:_____   Date:___Today___
Patient Address:_____   Age:_____

R_x

Tab Synthroid 75mcg
Sig: T PO EOD UD
#100

Refill: _3_

Hahneman Family Clinic
Dr. C.C. Egbus, M.D
158 95th Avenue Bearspaw Ranchlands
Northwest Calgary, AB. T0Y 5N7
Phone: 403 103 2359

Patient Name:_____   Date:___Today___
Patient Address:_____   Age:_____

R_x

Levemir Insulin 100 units/ml
Sig: Inj. 38 units SC QPM UD
M: 45ml

Refill: _Ø_

DR. JOE KINGSON, M.D, F.R.C.P
Jophil Medical Clinic
Fountain Plaza, 54 Broadstreet SW,
Calgary, AB. T3X OP3
Phone: 587 724 1193

Patient Name:_____   Date: Today

Patient Address:_____   Age:_____

R$_x$

TAB. FOSAMAX 70MG

Sig: T PO QWEEK 2HR AC UD

M: 4 TABS

Refill: 12

Hahneman Family Clinic
Dr. C.C. Egbus, M.D
158 95th Avenue Bearspaw Ranchlands
Northwest Calgary, AB. T0Y 5N7
Phone: 403 103 2359

Patient Name:_____   Date: Totay

Patient Address:_____   Age:_____

R$_x$

Ventolin Inhaler 100µg

Sig: ii puffs Q4-6H PRN SOB

#1

Refill: Ø

DR. JOE KINGSON, M.D, F.R.C.P
Jophil Medical Clinic
Fountain Plaza, 54 Broadstreet SW,
Calgary, AB. T3X OP3
Phone: 587 724 1193

Patient Name:_____   Date: __Today____
Patient Address:_____   Age:_____

R_x

TAB LASIX 40mg
SIG: Ṫ QAM @ 800 PRN
M: 100 TABS

Refill: Ø

Hahneman Family Clinic
Dr. C.C. Egbus, M.D
158 95th Avenue Bearspaw Ranchlands
Northwest Calgary, AB. T0Y 5N7
Phone: 403 103 2359

Patient Name:_____   Date: __Today____
Patient Address:_____   Age:_____

R_x

Nitroglycerin SL Spray
Sig: Ṫ Spray SL Q5min Max 3 doses
                                    PRN
M: One Bottle

Refill: Ø

⑱

DR. JOE KINGSON, M.D, F.R.C.P
Jophil Medical Clinic
Fountain Plaza, 54 Broadstreet SW,
Calgary, AB. T3X OP3
Phone: 587 724 1193

Patient Name:_____   Date:___Today_____

Patient Address:_____   Age:_____

R

Zithromex swp 10 mg/kg/day
po 1ˢᵗ day + 5 mg/kg/day po
next 4 days (wt 12.5 kgs

Refill:___∅___

Hahneman Family Clinic
⑲
Dr. C.C. Egbus, M.D
158 95th Avenue Bearspaw Ranchlands
Northwest Calgary, AB. T0Y 5N7
Phone: 403 103 2359

Patient Name:_____   Date:___Today_____

Patient Address:_____   Age:_____

R

Tetracycline Caps 250mg
Sig: 4 caps PO BID D/c after 5 days UD

#40 Capsules

Refill:___∅___

20

DR. JOE KINGSON, M.D, F.R.C.P

Jophil Medical Clinic

Fountain Plaza, 54 Broadstreet SW,
Calgary, AB. T3X OP3
Phone: 587 724 1193

Patient Name:_____   Date: Today_____

Patient Address:_____   Age:_____

R_x

Nix Cream Rinse
Sig: AAA Nocte, Leave for 24 hrs UD
#80 grams

Refill:_____

21

Hahneman Family Clinic

Dr. C.C. Egbus, M.D

158 95th Avenue Bearspaw Ranchlands
Northwest Calgary, AB. T0Y 5N7
Phone: 403 103 2359

Patient Name:_____   Date: Today_____

Patient Address:_____   Age:_____

R_x

Gtt Nigamox ophth.
Sig: T. Gtt OU TID UD
M: 3 mL

Refill: Ø

DR. JOE KINGSON, M.D, F.R.C.P
Jophil Medical Clinic
Fountain Plaza, 54 Broadstreet SW,
Calgary, AB. T3X OP3
Phone: 587 724 1193

Patient Name:_____   Date: Today_____

Patient Address:_____   Age:_____

R_x

Tab clonazepam 2mg

Sig: ss — ī tab PO Q6-8H & QHS PRN anxiety.

Supply 30 tabs   Refill: Ø

Hahneman Family Clinic
Dr. C.C. Egbus, M.D
158 95th Avenue Bearspaw Ranchlands
Northwest Calgary, AB. T0Y 5N7
Phone: 403 103 2359

Patient Name:_____   Date: Today_____

Patient Address:_____   Age:_____

R_x

Ciprodex Otic

Sig: IV gtt AD QID PRN

M: 7.5mL

Refill: Ø

DR. JOE KINGSON, M.D, F.R.C.P
Jophil Medical Clinic
Fountain Plaza, 54 Broadstreet SW,
Calgary, AB. T3X OP3
Phone: 587 724 1193

Patient Name:_____

Patient Address:_____

Date: __Today__

Age:_____

R

Victoza 0.6mg S/C OD x 1/52

~~then~~ 1.2mg S/C OD x 3/12

Refill:___1___

Hahneman Family Clinic
Dr. C.C. Egbus, M.D
158 95th Avenue Bearspaw Ranchlands
Northwest Calgary, AB. T0Y 5N7
Phone: 403 103 2359

Patient Name:_____

Patient Address:_____

Date: __Today__

Age:_____

R

Elix. Cotridine Expt.

Sig: Take 2 tsp HS PRN Cough

M: 100ml

Refill:___∅___

(26)

DR. JOE KINGSON, M.D, F.R.C.P
Jophil Medical Clinic
Fountain Plaza, 54 Broadstreet SW,
Calgary, AB. T3X OP3
Phone: 587 724 1193

Patient Name:_____   Date: _Today_

Patient Address:_____   Age:_____

R_x

Tab Zithromax (Z-pack) 250mg
Sig: ïï PO stat for day 1
Then ī PO QD for days 2–5
    Supply 6 tablets   Refill:__Ø__

---

(27)

Hahneman Family Clinic
Dr. C.C. Egbus, M.D
158 95th Avenue Bearspaw Ranchlands
Northwest Calgary, AB. T0Y 5N7
Phone: 403 103 2359

Patient Name:_____   Date: _Today_

Patient Address:_____   Age:_____

R_x

Novolin Insulin GE
Sig: Inj. 35 Units SC 15mins AC
    3/12

                                        Refill:__Ø__

DR. JOE KINGSON, M.D, F.R.C.P
Jophil Medical Clinic
Fountain Plaza, 54 Broadstreet SW,
Calgary, AB. T3X OP3
Phone: 587 724 1193

Patient Name:_____ Date: _Today_____

Patient Address:_____ Age:_____

R_x

Tab metoprolol 50mg
Sig: T PO QD if BP > 140/85
#30

Refill: ∅

Hahneman Family Clinic

Dr. C.C. Egbus, M.D
158 95th Avenue Bearspaw Ranchlands
Northwest Calgary, AB. T0Y 5N7
Phone: 403 103 2359

Patient Name:_____ Date: _Today_____

Patient Address:_____ Age:_____

R_x

Levofloxacin 500mg po
x one
then 250 mg po od
x 7d.

Refill: Zero

(30)

DR. JOE KINGSON, M.D, F.R.C.P
Jophil Medical Clinic
Fountain Plaza, 54 Broadstreet SW,
Calgary, AB. T3X OP3
Phone: 587 724 1193

Patient Name:_____

Patient Address:_____

Date:___Today___

Age:_____

R̲

Com Hydeum
Sig: Apply approx 2g face PRN uD
M: 100 grams

Refill:___∅___

---

(31)

Hahneman Family Clinic
Dr. C.C. Egbus, M.D
158 95th Avenue Bearspaw Ranchlands
Northwest Calgary, AB. T0Y 5N7
Phone: 403 103 2359

Patient Name:_____

Patient Address:_____

Date:___Today___

Age:_____

R̲

R Doxycycline 100mg
2 tabs PO day 1
then 1 tab PO BID
days 2 - 14

Refill:___∅___

191

DR. JOE KINGSON, M.D, F.R.C.P
Jophil Medical Clinic
Fountain Plaza, 54 Broadstreet SW,
Calgary, AB. T3X OP3
Phone: 587 724 1193

Patient Name:_____

Patient Address:_____

Date: Today

Age:_____

Rx

Ung. Dermovate

AAA Top. BID PRN

60 grams

Refill: Ø

Hahneman Family Clinic
Dr. C.C. Egbus, M.D
158 95th Avenue Bearspaw Ranchlands
Northwest Calgary, AB. T0Y 5N7
Phone: 403 103 2359

Patient Name:_____

Patient Address:_____

Date: Today

Age:_____

Rx

Septra DS

i̅ B ID

M: 20 tabs

Refill: Ø

(34)

DR. JOE KINGSON, M.D, F.R.C.P
Jophil Medical Clinic
Fountain Plaza, 54 Broadstreet SW,
Calgary, AB. T3X OP3
Phone: 587 724 1193

Patient Name:_____ Date: Today

Patient Address:_____ Age:_____

R

Zantac Liq. 15mg/ml
Sig: ii tbsp cc lunch PRN
M: 100ml

Refill: Ø

(35)

Hahneman Family Clinic
Dr. C.C. Egbus, M.D
158 95th Avenue Bearspaw Ranchlands
Northwest Calgary, AB. T0Y 5N7
Phone: 403 103 2359

Patient Name:_____ Date: Today

Patient Address:_____ Age:_____

R

Gtt. Tobradex ophth.
Sig: ii Gtt BID OD uD 10/7
Supply One Bottle

Refill: Ø

DR. JOE KINGSON, M.D, F.R.C.P

Jophil Medical Clinic

Fountain Plaza, 54 Broadstreet SW,
Calgary, AB. T3X OP3
Phone: 587 724 1193

Patient Name:_____

Patient Address:_____

Date:_____Today_____

Age:_____

R_x

Tab Tylenol Regular 325mg
Sig: ⊤ — ⊤⊤ Q4-6H PRNP UD
M: 100 tabs

Refill:_____∅_____

Hahneman Family Clinic

Dr. C.C. Egbus, M.D

158 95th Avenue Bearspaw Ranchlands
Northwest Calgary, AB. T0Y 5N7
Phone: 403 103 2359

Patient Name:_____

Patient Address:_____

Date:_____Today_____

Age:_____

R_x

Tab atwan 1mg SL
Sig: 1 SL 1 Hr prior to Appt UD
#2

Refill:___3___

(38) DR. JOE KINGSON, M.D, F.R.C.P
Jophil Medical Clinic
Fountain Plaza, 54 Broadstreet SW,
Calgary, AB. T3X OP3
Phone: 587 724 1193

Patient Name:_____

Patient Address:_____

Date:___Today___

Age:_____

R_x

Ciprodex otic
Sig: IV gtt AU Q12H PRN
M: 7.5ml

Refill:___∅___

Hahneman Family Clinic
(39) Dr. C.C. Egbus, M.D
158 95th Avenue Bearspaw Ranchlands
Northwest Calgary, AB. T0Y 5N7
Phone: 403 103 2359

Patient Name:_____

Patient Address:_____

Date:___Today___

Age:_____

R_x

Amoxicillin liquid 250mg/5ml
Sig: 7.5ml PO TID for 10/7
Supp. liquid formulation only.

Refill:___∅___

195

DR. JOE KINGSON, M.D, F.R.C.P
Jophil Medical Clinic
Fountain Plaza, 54 Broadstreet SW,
Calgary, AB. T3X OP3
Phone: 587 724 1193

Patient Name:_____

Patient Address:_____

Date:____Today____

Age:_____

R_x

Twin Rix + IM injection @
days 0, 7 and 21
— accelerated dosing.

Refill:___∅___

Hahneman Family Clinic
Dr. C.C. Egbus, M.D
158 95th Avenue Bearspaw Ranchlands
Northwest Calgary, AB. T0Y 5N7
Phone: 403 103 2359

Patient Name:_____

Patient Address:_____

Date:____Today____

Age:_____

R_x

Amoxicillin 500mg Capsules
Sig: ii PO Q8H UF
1/52

Refill:___∅___

DR. JOE KINGSON, M.D, F.R.C.P
Jophil Medical Clinic
Fountain Plaza, 54 Broadstreet SW,
Calgary, AB. T3X OP3
Phone: 587 724 1193

Patient Name:_____ Date: Today_____
Patient Address:_____ Age:_____

R_x

Inj. Morphine Sulfate 5mg/2ml
Sig: 2ml IM QHS PRNP
M: 50ml

Refill: Ø

Hahneman Family Clinic
Dr. C.C. Egbus, M.D
158 95th Avenue Bearspaw Ranchlands
Northwest Calgary, AB. T0Y 5N7
Phone: 403 103 2359

Patient Name:_____ Date: Today_____
Patient Address:_____ Age:_____

R_x

Cerumol Otic
Sig: Gtt IV AS wax
M: 30ml

Refill: Ø

DR. JOE KINGSON, M.D, F.R.C.P
Jophil Medical Clinic
Fountain Plaza, 54 Broadstreet SW,
Calgary, AB. T3X OP3
Phone: 587 724 1193

Patient Name:_____ Date: Today_____

Patient Address:_____ Age:_____

Rx

Compound Diclofenac 12% in Difusimax
Sig: Apply QAM & QPM Knee (L) PRN
M: 150 gram

Refill: ∅

Hahneman Family Clinic

Dr. C.C. Egbus, M.D
158 95th Avenue Bearspaw Ranchlands
Northwest Calgary, AB. T0Y 5N7
Phone: 403 103 2359

Patient Name:_____ Date: Today_____

Patient Address:_____ Age:_____

Rx

Diclofenac gel 8%.

Apply to painful area ∅ prn.
    –bid ⇒ tid.
        Mitte: 200 grams

Refill: 2

(46)

DR. JOE KINGSON, M.D, F.R.C.P

Jophil Medical Clinic

Fountain Plaza, 54 Broadstreet SW,
Calgary, AB. T3X OP3
Phone: 587 724 1193

Patient Name:_____   Date:___Today___
Patient Address:_____   Age:_____

Rx

Tab prednisolone 5mg
Sig: 40 mg PO QD
Then ↓ by 5mg Q week
until done

Refill:___∅___

Hahneman Family Clinic

(47)

Dr. C.C. Egbus, M.D

158 95th Avenue Bearspaw Ranchlands
Northwest Calgary, AB. T0Y 5N7
Phone: 403 103 2359

Patient Name:_____   Date:___Today___
Patient Address:_____   Age:_____

Rx

Cap Flagyl 500mg
Sig: II Cap PO TID x 3wks
Then i Cap PO BID x 2wks
Then i Cap PO QD UF

#200 Caps   Refill:___∅___

DR. JOE KINGSON, M.D, F.R.C.P
Jophil Medical Clinic
Fountain Plaza, 54 Broadstreet SW,
Calgary, AB. T3X OP3
Phone: 587 724 1193

Patient Name:_____   Date: Today
Patient Address:_____   Age:_____

Rx

Imovane 7.5g

1-2 po qhs PRN

mitte: 100

Refill:___1

Hahneman Family Clinic

Dr. C.C. Egbus, M.D
158 95th Avenue Bearspaw Ranchlands
Northwest Calgary, AB. T0Y 5N7
Phone: 403 103 2359

Patient Name:_____   Date: Today
Patient Address:_____   Age:_____

Rx

Regular Insulin
Sig: 20 Units Sc QAM and
30 Units Sc 45mins Pc Lunch
#10ml Vial   Refill:___∅

DR. JOE KINGSON, M.D, F.R.C.P
Jophil Medical Clinic
Fountain Plaza, 54 Broadstreet SW,
Calgary, AB. T3X OP3
Phone: 587 724 1193

Patient Name:_____

Patient Address:_____

Date:___Today___

Age:_____

R_x

Tab Valtrex 500mg

Sig: 1 gram PO BID 3/7

PRN UD

12 tabs

Refill:___∅___

Answers to Chapter 5 Practice Questions

1. Take half a tablet orally daily if heart rate increases as directed (blood pressure / cardiac palpitation)

2. Take 250 mg three times daily for seven days (bacterial infection)

3. Take half a tablet orally every morning and one tablet orally at bedtime as needed (insomnia)

4. Take two tablets once daily until finished (bacterial infection)

5. Take one tablet orally every four to six hours as needed for pain (pain and inflammation)

6. Take one tablet orally twice daily with food as needed (pain and inflammation)

7. Inject 0.65 mL subcutaneously at once as directed (vaccination against shingles)

8. Take two tablets orally every two to four hours after meals as needed for painful gout (acute gouty arthritis)

9. Take one or two tablets orally every four to six hours as needed (pain)

10. Apply one strip to the lower eyelid of the left eye twice daily (bacterial eye infection)

11. Insert one suppository rectally at night as directed (hemorrhoid)

12. Take one tablet orally every other day as directed (hypothyroidism)

13. Inject 38 units subcutaneously every evening as directed (diabetes)

14. Take one tablet orally every week, two hours before meals as directed (osteoporosis)

15. Inhale two puffs every four to six hours as needed for shortness of breath (asthma reliever)

16. Take one tablet every morning at 8 a.m. as needed (diuresis, edema, or blood pressure)

17. Use one spray under the tongue every five minutes for a maximum of three doses as needed (angina pectoris)

18. Take 125 mg orally for day 1 and then take 62.5 mg orally once daily for next four days (bacterial infection)

19. Take four capsules orally twice daily, discontinue after five days as directed (bacterial infection)

20. Apply to affected area at night, leave in place for twenty-four hours, as directed

21. Instill one drop into both eyes three times daily as directed (bacterial eye infection)

22. Take half or one tablet orally every six to eight hours and every bedtime as needed (anxiety)

23. Instill four drops into the right ear four times daily as needed (ear infection and inflammation)

24. Inject 0.6 mg subcutaneously once daily for one week, then 1.2 mg subcutaneously once daily for three months (diabetes)

25. Take two teaspoonfuls at bedtime as needed for cough (cough and removal of sputum)

26. Take two tablets orally at once for day 1, then take one tablet orally once daily for days 2–5 (bacterial infection)

27. Inject 35 units subcutaneously fifteen minutes before meals (diabetes)

28. Take one tablet orally once daily if blood pressure is greater than 140/85 (blood pressure)

29. Take two tablets (500 mg) at once, then take one tablet (250 mg) orally once daily for seven days (bacterial infection)

30. Apply approximately 2 g to face as needed as directed (eczema, skin reactions)

31. Take two tablets orally for day 1, then take one tablet orally twice daily for days 2–14 (bacterial infection)

32. Apply to affected area topically twice daily as needed (psoriasis, eczema, or skin reactions)

33. Take one tablet twice daily (bacterial infection)

34. Take two tablespoonfuls with lunch as needed (ulcer or gastric reflux disorder)

35. Instill two drops into the right eye twice daily as directed for ten days (eye bacterial inflammatory condition)

36. Take one or two tablets every four to six hours as needed for pain as directed (pain)

37. Dissolve one tablet under the tongue one hour prior to dental appointment as directed (anxiety)

38. Instill four drops into both ears every twelve hours as needed (ear infection and inflammation)

39. Give 7.5 mL orally three times daily for ten days only. Supply only liquid amoxicillin (bacterial infection)

40. For intramuscular injection at days 0, 7, and 21—accelerated dosing schedule (Hepatitis A and B vaccination)

41. Take two capsules orally every eight hours until finished (bacterial infection)

42. Inject 2 mL intramuscularly daily at bedtime as needed for pain (pain relief)

43. Instill four drops into the left ear for wax removal (wax build up in the ear)

44. Apply every morning and every evening to left knee as needed (pain and inflammation)

45. Apply to painful area as needed twice to three times daily (pain and inflammation)

46. Take eight tablets orally once daily then decrease by one tablet every week until done (inflammation)

47. Take two capsules orally three times daily for three weeks, then take one capsule twice daily for two weeks, then take one capsule orally once daily until finished

48. Take one or two tablets orally daily at bedtime as needed (insomnia or for sleep)

49. Inject 20 units subcutaneously every morning and 30 units subcutaneously forty-five minutes after lunch

50. Take two tablets (1,000 mg) orally twice daily for three days as needed as directed (viral infection)

CHAPTER 6

Dosage Calculations

Objectives

At the end of this chapter, students should be able to do the following:

- Differentiate between single dose, daily dose, and total dose
- Demonstrate understanding of the full content of a medication order
- Calculate the total quantity ordered in a medication order/ prescription
- Determine the appropriate duration of a prescription
- Perform simple dosage calculations

The dose of a drug is the quantity of medication administered or consumed by the patient for the intended therapeutic effect. It is important to understand that some drugs, by their nature, are only consumed once; others are also consumed several times a day for only a few days; and some are consumed once or several times a day for several days. Based on this, the dose of a drug can be distinguished as either single dose, daily dose, or total dose.

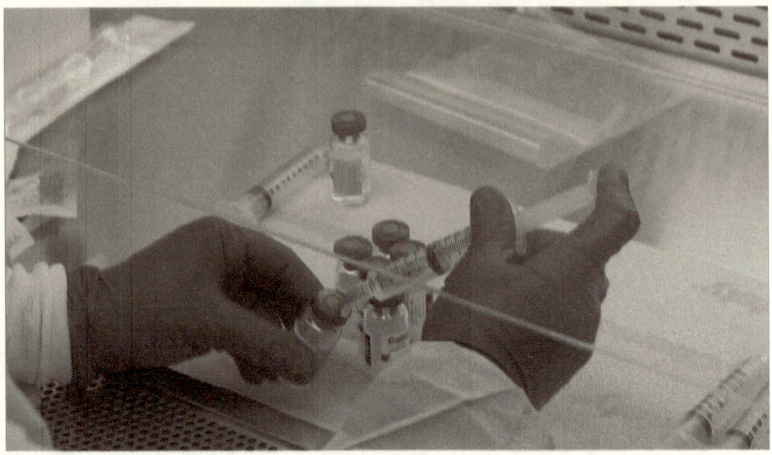

FIGURE 6.1 *Reconstitution and Withdrawal of Liquid Medication from Vials:* When withdrawing a specified amount of medication from a vial, guided by the labelled strength of the formulation, a professional must ensure the withdrawn volume contains the defined amount of the active ingredient in accordance with the prescription.

Single dose is the amount of drug taken or administered at *one time.* "One time" means how much of the medication is put in the mouth (or administered through other routes) at one time. For example, consider the prescription

> Biaxin XL 500 mg
>
> Sig: ii po once daily $\dfrac{10}{7}$

The single dose of the Biaxin XL as prescribed above is two tablets or 1,000 mg because the patient will be required to take two tablets per single consumption. The instruction above is quite different from the one below:

> Biaxin 500 mg
>
> Sig: i po BID $\dfrac{10}{7}$

Although in both cases the patient will ultimately consume two tablets per day and twenty tablets in ten days, the single doses are different. It's two tablets for Biaxin XL but only one tablet for Biaxin regular.

Daily dose is the amount of medication that is administered in one full day (twenty-four-hour full day). One day is considered to be a period of twenty-four hours. Consider the prescription:

Amoxicillin 500 mg

Sig: i po TID $\dfrac{10}{7}$

The daily dose of the amoxicillin is

1 × 3 = 3 capsules or 1,500 mg

because the patient is required to take 500 mg three times daily.

Consider the following prescription:

Biaxin 500 mg XL

Sig: ii po once daily $\dfrac{10}{7}$

The daily dose is two tablets = 1,000 mg, which, in this case, is also the single dose.

Consider the following prescription:

Tylenol #3
Sig: ii Q8H PRN
    M: 100

The sig of the prescription can be interpreted as this: "Take two tablets every eight hours as needed." It should be noted that taking the medication every eight hours is equivalent to taking the medication three times in twenty-four hours (because one day is twenty-four hours).

$$24 \text{ hrs} \div 8 = 3 \text{ times}$$

So the daily dosage is 2 tablets × 3 = 6 tablets. On the other hand, if a prescription is written for Q6H, this is taken to mean four times daily because 24 hrs ÷ 6 = 4 times.

The following table will serve as a guide in the calculation of daily doses.

Frequency	Interpretation
Q1H	24 times daily
Q2H	12 times daily
Q3H	8 times daily
Q4H	6 times daily
Q6H	4 times daily
Q8H	3 times daily
Q12H	2 times daily
Q24H	Once daily

Note: For prescriptions whose dosage is written as a range (for example i or ii tablets daily), our single and daily dose calculations must be based on the maximum amount of medication consumable from the prescription as written.

For example,

Tylenol Regular (325 mg)

Sig: i–ii tablets TID PRN

M: 100

The prescription reads 'one or two tablets three times daily as needed'. Patient has the option of taking one or two tablets as a single dose, but our calculation of a daily dose should be based on two tablets three times daily, which means patient can take a maximum of 2 tablets as single dose and a maximum of six tablets daily.

Consider the prescription:

> Tylenol Extra Strength
> Sig: i–ii tablets Q4-6H PRN
>
> $$\frac{10}{7}$$

Here the patient has the option of taking one or two tablets as a single dose and also has the option of taking the single dose every four hours or every six hours as needed.

The highest amount of single dose is two tablets (as two is greater than one), and the highest frequency of consumption is every four hours because the patient will consume more drugs every four hours (six times a day) than every six hours (four times a day). Hence, to calculate our daily dose, it should be based on two tablets every four hours, which is

$$2 \times 6 = 12 \text{ tablets (maximum per day)}$$

Therefore, for the prescription above, the total dose should be calculated based on twelve tablets daily.

Total dose of a drug is the total amount of medication consumed during the course of the therapy. The schedule of dosing (for example, amoxicillin 500 mg TID for seven days) is referred to as the dosage regimen. In this case, the total dose of the amoxicillin will be twenty-one capsules of the 500 mg strength.

The total dose of a drug can be provided by the prescriber in two different ways.

In prescription writing, the prescriber can directly indicate the total quantity of medication prescribed in the prescription or alternatively indicate the number of days the medication should be consumed.

For example,

> Penicillin VK 300 mg
>
> Sig: ii po TID UF
>
> 60 tablets

Here the total dose is sixty tablets. In this case, the pharmacy professional will have the responsibility of assigning the duration (the number of days) of the therapy.

In the example above, the single dose is two tablets, the daily dose is six tablets, and the duration of therapy is ten days.

On the other hand, the prescriber can indirectly indicate the total dose by specifying the number of days of therapy.

For example,

> Colchicine 0.1 mg
>
> i–ii tablets Q12H PRN
>
> M: 10 days

The single dose of the medication is one or two tablets, but we will use two tablets in our calculation because two is the maximum single dose. The daily dose will be 2 tablets × 2 = 4 tablets. (Q12H means two times in twenty-four hours.) Total dose of the prescription will be 2 × 2 × 10 = 40 tablets.

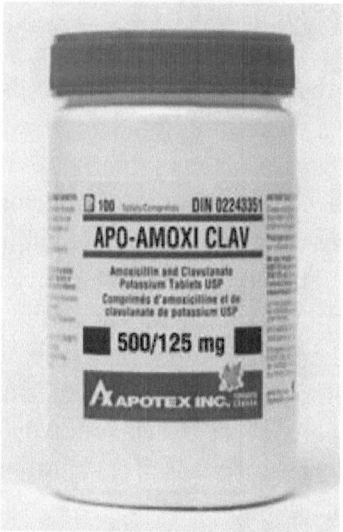

FIGURE 6.2 ***Multiple Therapeutic Ingredient Tablet:*** Some tablets contain
more than one relevant therapeutic ingredient. When calculating doses,
these ingredients must be taken into consideration to ensure that patients
are receiving the exact amounts of the ingredients prescribed. Each tablet
of the Apo-Amoxicillin/Clavulanic acid shown above contains 500 mg of
amoxicillin and 125 mg of clavulanic acid. The two ingredients act through
synergy to produce a better outcome in battling some bacterial infection.

Teaspoon and Tablespoon

In calculating doses, pharmacists and physicians/prescribers accept a
capacity of *5 mL* for a teaspoonful and *15 mL* for a tablespoonful. The
teaspoons available in our individual household may not necessarily
deliver 5 mL of medication but may deliver liquids in the range of 3 to 7
mL. In the same way, the tablespoons in the house may deliver liquids in
the range of 15 to 22 mL. Hence, when instructing patients on dosages
written in teaspoons or tablespoons, patients must be specifically
advised on the exact amount to administer because different cultures
have different concepts of teaspoons and tablespoons. Therefore,

1 teaspoonful (tsp) = 5 mL

1 tablespoonful (tbsp) = 15 mL

The Drop as a Unit of Measure

Sometimes medications such as eye drops, ear drops, and some liquid oral formulations, like vitamin D liquid and nystatin suspension, are prescribed in unit doses of drops (abbreviated as *gtt*). It should be noted that a drop doesn't represent a definite volume of fluid because the volume that makes up a drop of different liquids vary greatly. The volume of a drop depends on: (1) the viscosity of the liquid, (2) the diameter of the dropper orifice from which the liquid drops, and (3) some other factors like temperature, pressure, and specific gravity of the liquid. In an attempt to standardize the drop as a dosage unit, a standard dropper is considered to release 20 drops per 1 mL of liquid from the dropper. For the purposes of calculations involving the drop, it is acceptable to consider

20 drops = 1 mL

1 mL = 20 drops

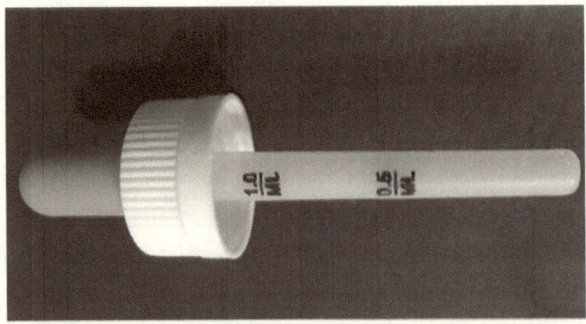

FIGURE 6.3 *The Calibrated Dropper:* This calibrated dropper is used for the oral administration of some liquid formulation (suspension, solution, elixir) to both adult and pediatric patients.

The Concept of Refills

When a prescription is written and refill is indicated, the prescriber's intention is that the prescription can be repeated the number of times indicated by the refill value.

For example, consider the following prescription:

> Rx
>
> Amlodipine 10 mg tablets
>
> Sig: i po qd for 30 days
>
> > × 5 refills

What the prescription is saying here is that after the first thirty days' supply from the prescription, the patient can receive another thirty days' supply for five times. Therefore, the total authorized quantity of the prescription is 180 tablets (that is, 30 plus [30 × 5] = 180). For new students in the health profession, there is the temptation of wrongly assuming that the total authorized quantity of the above prescription is 30 × 5. The total authorized quantity of the prescription is rather 30 × 6 = 180 tablets. It is worth noting that we add one to the number of refills indicated before we multiply by a one-time authorized quantity.

Consider this prescription:

> Rx
>
> Metoprolol 25 mg
>
> Sig: i BID for 90 days
>
> > × 2 refills

The one-time authorized fill is 180 tablets for 90 days.

The total authorized quantity in the prescription is 180 × (2 + 1) = 540 tablets.

Example 6.1

Consider the following prescription:

> Metoprolol 25 mg
>
> Sig: ii po BID 100 days

(a) What is the single dose in milligrams?
(b) What is the daily dose in milligrams?
(c) What is the total dose in milligrams?

Solution

(a) Single dose is

$$2 \text{ tablets of } 25 \text{ mg} = 50 \text{ mg}$$

(b) Daily dose is

$$2 \text{ tablets of } 25 \text{ mg} \times 2$$
$$= 50 \text{ mg} \times 2$$
$$= 100 \text{ mg}$$

(c) Total dose is

$$2 \times 2 \times 100 = 400 \text{ tablets}$$
$$= 400 \times 25 \text{ mg}$$
$$= 10,000 \text{ mg}$$

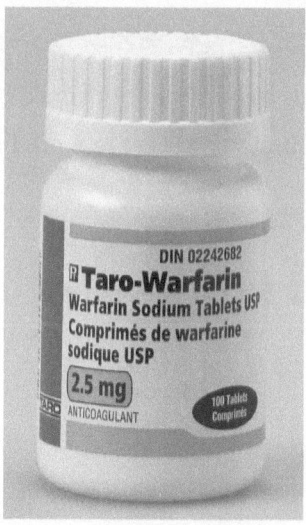

FIGURE 6.4 *Taro-Warfarin 2.5 mg Tablets:* Each tablet contains 2.5 mg of the active ingredient warfarin. If a prescription calls for 1.25 mg of warfarin once daily, then half of this tablet should be administered daily. If the prescription calls for 5 mg warfarin once daily and only 2.5 mg strength is available, then 2 tablets of this should be administered daily. (Courtesy Taro pharmaceuticals)

Example 6.2

Referring to example 6.1 above, if metoprolol is only available as 50 mg tablets,

    (a) What is the single dose in number of tablets?
    (b) What is the daily dose in number of tablets?
    (c) What is the total dose in number of tablets?

Solution

    (a) From the prescription, single dose is 2 tablets of 25 mg = 50 mg

        If the available strength is 50 mg tablets, then one tablet should be administered. So the single dose is one tablet of 50 mg.

(b) Daily dose will be

Single dose × number of times per day

1 tablet × 2 = 2 tablets of 50mg

(c) Total dose will be

Single dose × number of times per day × number of days

$$= 1 \times 2 \times 100$$

$$= 200 \text{ tablets}$$

Example 6.3

Consider the following prescription:

Rx

Acetaminophen Regular Strength (325 mg)

Sig: ii–iii PO QID PRN

M: 120 tablets

(a) What is the maximum single dose?
(b) What is the maximum daily dose?
(c) What will be the duration assigned to the prescription?

Solution

(a) The single dose is two or three tablets; therefore, the maximum single dose is 3 tablets.

(b) Maximum daily dose is

Maximum single dose × number of times per day

$$= 3 \times 4 = 12 \text{ tablets}$$

(c) The duration of therapy

$$12 \text{ tablets} \rightarrow 1 \text{ day}$$

$$120 \text{ tablets} \rightarrow u$$

$$u = \frac{1 \ day}{12 \ tablets} \times \frac{120 \ tablets}{1}$$

$$= 10 \text{ days}$$

Example 6.4

Consider the following prescription:

Ibuprofen 200 mg

Sig: i–ii tablets Q6-8H PRN

3/52

(a) What is the maximum single dose?
(b) What is the maximum daily dose?
(c) How many tablets should be dispensed for the entire duration (3 /52 = 3 weeks = 21 days) of the therapy?

Solution

(a) Single dose is 1 or 2 tablets, but the maximum single dose is 2 tablets
(b) Maximum daily dose is

Maximum single dose × maximum number of times per day

$$= 2 \times 4 \text{ (Q6H means 4} \times \text{per day)}$$

$$= 2 \times 4 = 8 \text{ tablets}$$

(c) Now the patient takes 8 tablets in a day, so we can say

$$1 \text{ day} \rightarrow 8 \text{ tablets}$$

$$21 \text{ days} \rightarrow u$$

$$u = \frac{8 \; tablets}{1 \; day} \times \frac{21 \; days}{1}$$

$$= 168 \text{ tablets}$$

Note: In dosage calculations, once we can figure out the daily dose, it will then be very easy to calculate the total quantity of medication for a given number of days, as well as calculate the duration of the therapy given the quantity of medication to be dispensed using any of these lines of proportion:

$$Q \rightarrow 1 \text{ day}$$

or

$$1 \text{ day} \rightarrow Q,$$

$$Q = \text{Quantity of medication}$$

Use the first if calculating the number of days.

Use the second if calculating the quantity of medication.

Example 6.5

Consider the following prescription:

Rx

Cephalexin 250 mg / 5 mL

Give 400 mg PO TID 10/7

Dispense liquid cephalexin only

(a) What is the single dose in milliliters?
(b) What is the daily dose in milliliters?
(c) How many milliliters will the patient consume for the duration?
(d) If cephalexin comes in unit bottles of 75 mL, 100 mL, and 150 mL, suggest the best possible pack size combination to be given to the patient that will make the most economic sense.

(e) Write out the correct instruction on the label for the patient.

(f) What amount of cephalexin in grams will the patient consume throughout the therapy?

Solution

(a) We apply proportion everywhere in pharmacy. An amount of 400 mg was prescribed as a single dose. The question is, what volume of the suspension will deliver 400 mg of cephalexin?

We use our proportion,

$$250 \text{ mg cephalexin} \rightarrow 5 \text{ mL suspension}$$
$$400 \text{ mg cephalexin} \rightarrow u$$
$$u = \frac{5 \ mL \ suspension}{250 \ mg \ cephalexin} \times \frac{400 \ mg \ cephalexin}{1}$$
$$= 8 \text{ mL}$$

Therefore, single dose = 8 mL.

(b) Daily dose is

$$\text{Single dose} \times \text{number of times per day}$$
$$= 8 \text{ mL} \times 3 = 24 \text{ mL}$$

(c) Total dose is

$$\text{Single dose} \times \text{number of times a day} \times \text{number of days}$$
$$[8 \text{ mL} \times 3] \times 10$$
$$= 240 \text{ mL}$$

(d) The best possible pack sizes to dispense to the patient will be

$$1 \text{ bottle of 150 mL} + 1 \text{ bottle of 100 mL}$$
$$= \text{total 250 mL}$$

Patient will discard only 10 mL at the end of the dosage regimen (which makes economic sense)

(e) The correct instruction to be given to the patient will read

"Give 8 mL three times daily for 10 days then
discard the remaining portion."

(f) To calculate the amount of cephalexin (in grams) that the patient will consume for the entire duration, we can do this in one of two ways.

We can go directly:

$$\text{single dose} = 400 \text{ mg}$$

$$\text{daily dose} = 400 \text{ mg} \times 3 = 1{,}200 \text{ mg}$$

$$\text{total dose} = 1{,}200 \times 10 = 12{,}000 \text{ mg} = 12 \text{ g}$$

Or we can get the amount through the total volume consumed.

Total volume consumed is 240 mL

But every 5 mL contains 250 mg cephalexin, so

5 mL suspension → 250 mg cephalexin

240 mL suspension → u

$$u = \frac{250 \text{ mg cephalexin}}{5 \text{ mL suspension}} \times \frac{240 \text{ mL suspension}}{1}$$

$$= 12{,}000 \text{ mg } or \text{ } 12 \text{ g}$$

Example 6.6

The dosage of a certain liquid cough medication, Robitussin, is 1 teaspoon three times daily. If 1 bottle of Robitussin is 200 mL, how long will one bottle last for a patient if the patient takes it as prescribed?

Solution

One teaspoon is 5 mL.

Dosage is 5 mL × 3 = 15 mL per day.

So daily dosage is 15 mL.

We can solve by proportion

$$15 \text{ mL} \rightarrow 1 \text{ day}$$
$$200 \text{ mL} \rightarrow u$$
$$U = \frac{1 \, day}{15 \, mL} \times \frac{200 \, mL}{1}$$
$$= 13.33 \text{ days}$$
Approx 13 days

Example 6.7

Consider the following prescription:

Gtt. Pred Forte 1%

Sig: Instill i gtt OU BID UD

M: 1 bottle of 5 mL

How long will the 5 mL bottle last for the patient if the patient uses the eye drop as prescribed?

Solution

The interpretation of the signature is as follows:

Instill one drop into both eyes twice daily as directed

Dispense 5 mL

Both eyes of the patient receive one drop each at one time, and this is done twice daily. So in one day, the patient uses four drops.

So daily dosage = 4 drops.

Now

$$1 \text{ mL} \rightarrow 20 \text{ drops}$$
$$5 \text{ mL} \rightarrow u$$
$$u = \frac{20 \text{ drops}}{1 \text{ mL}} \times \frac{5 \text{ mL}}{1}$$
$$= 100 \text{ drops}$$

So there are 100 drops in a 5 mL bottle

But

$$4 \text{ drops are used in 1 day.}$$

So

$$4 \text{ drops} \rightarrow 1 \text{ day}$$
$$100 \text{ drops} \rightarrow u$$
$$u = \frac{1 \text{ day}}{4 \text{ drops}} \times \frac{100 \text{ drops}}{1}$$
$$= 25 \text{ days}$$

Therefore, the 5 mL will last the patient 25 days.

Example 6.8

If a single dose of a drug is 200 mg, how many doses will be contained in 10 g?

Solution

Using our proportion,

$$200 \text{ mg} \rightarrow 1 \text{ dose}$$
$$10 \text{ g} \rightarrow u$$

Realize that the units on the left are not the same even though they are measures of weight. Therefore, the 10 g needs to be converted to milligrams to make both units of weight the same. (See chapter 2 for interconversion of units.)

$$1 \text{ g} \rightarrow 1,000 \text{ mg}$$
$$10 \text{ g} \rightarrow u$$

$$u = \frac{1,000 \text{ mg}}{1 \text{ g}} \times \frac{10 \text{ g}}{1}$$

$$= 10,000 \text{ mg}$$

Continuing

$$200 \text{ mg} \rightarrow 1 \text{ dose}$$
$$10,000 \text{ mg} \rightarrow u$$

$$u = \frac{1 \text{ dose}}{200 \text{ mg}} \times \frac{10,000 \text{ mg}}{1}$$

$$= 100 \text{ doses}$$

Example 6.9

If one teaspoon of a medication is prescribed as a single dose of a liquid medication, approximately how many doses will be contained in two cups?

Solution

$$1 \text{ teaspoon} = 5 \text{ mL}$$

Using proportion, we can say

$$5 \text{ mL} \rightarrow 1 \text{ dose}$$
$$2 \text{ cups} \rightarrow u$$

The units on the left (mL and cup) are not the same, so the cup needs to be converted to milliliters so both can be the same unit.

$$1 \text{ cup} \rightarrow 240 \text{ mL}$$
$$2 \text{ cups} \rightarrow u$$

$$u = \frac{240 \ mL}{1 \ cup} \times \frac{2 \ cups}{1}$$

$$= 480 \text{ mL}$$

Continuing

$$5 \text{ mL} \rightarrow 1 \text{ dose}$$
$$480 \text{ mL} \rightarrow u$$

$$u = \frac{1 \ dose}{5 \ mL} \times \frac{480 \ mL}{1}$$

$$= 96 \text{ doses}$$

Example 6.10

If 200 mL of Buckley's cough syrup contains 50 doses of the medication, what volume in milliliters is equivalent to 4 doses?

Solution

$$50 \text{ doses} \rightarrow 200 \text{ mL}$$
$$4 \text{ doses} \rightarrow u$$

$$u = \frac{200 \; mL}{50 \; doses} \times \frac{4 \; doses}{1}$$

$$= 16 \text{ mL}$$

Example 6.11

How many milliliters of a liquid medication would provide a physician with 2 tbsp TID for fourteen days?

Solution

$$2 \text{ tbsp} = 2 \times 15$$

$$= 30 \text{ mL}$$

Total mL prescribed is

$$30 \text{ mL} \times 3 \times 14$$

$$= 1,260 \text{ mL}$$

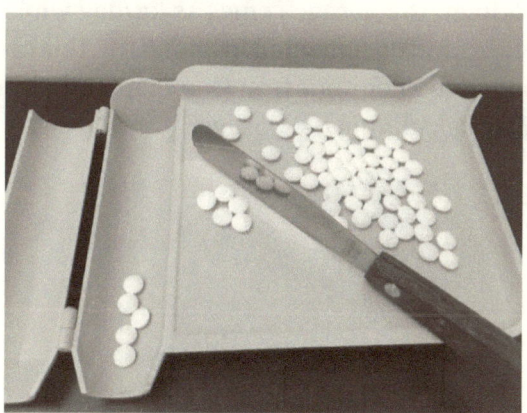

FIGURE 6.5 *The Counting Tray:* Solid oral dosage forms such as tablets and capsules should be accurately counted using the spatula and counting tray and never with the bare hands. It is conventional to count by 5's for better accuracy and speed of counting. Some pharmacies now use automatic counting machines to count their tablets and capsules.

Dosage Calculation Based on Body Parameters

Sometimes the dosage of medication for children and the elderly or other patients in special population are based on their body parameters. Children, especially, have unique body compositions that are different than those of adults. This unique body composition affects both the pharmacokinetics (what the body does to the drug) and pharmacodynamics (what the drug does to the body) of administered drugs. Pediatric and geriatric prescribers are always conscious of this very fact. In order to accommodate the varying ranges of dosages possible in these special populations, physicians mostly prescribe pediatric/geriatric medications based on

- body weight,
- body surface area (BSA), *or*
- age.

In pharmacy, we mainly encounter pediatric dosages based on weight, and this will form the focus of our discussion in this part of the chapter. Most times, the dosage comes as kg/day while the patient's weight is provided and documented in pounds. In this case, we need to convert the pound to kilograms first (see chapter 2, "Interconversion of Units") before calculating the dosage.

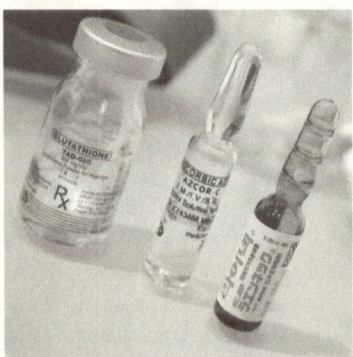

FIGURE 6.6 *Ampoules and Vials:* From L-R Vial, ampoule, ampoule. Some liquid medications, especially injectables, are packaged in ampoules or vials with a labelled concentration such that a specific volume of the liquid formulation (or product of reconstitution) will contain a defined amount of the active ingredient.

Example 6.12

Consider this prescription for pediatric ranitidine liquid:

> Rx
>
> Ranitidine 4 mg/kg/day every 24 hours for 30 days

Ranitidine comes in the strength 15 mg/mL

Patient weighs 34.95 kg.

(a) Calculate the daily dosage in milliliters.
(b) Calculate the total authorized volume to be dispensed to the patient for 30 days.
(c) Calculate the amount of ranitidine in milligrams that will be consumed by the patient at the end of the 30 days.

Solution

(a) First get the amount of ranitidine in milligrams that is the desired dosage.

An amount of 4 mg/kg/day means that every 1 kg body weight of the child receives 4 mg of ranitidine.

$$1 \text{ kg body weight} \rightarrow 4 \text{ mg}$$
$$34.95 \text{ kg body weight} \rightarrow u$$

$$u = \frac{4 \text{ mg}}{1 \text{ kg}} \times \frac{34.95 \text{ kg}}{1}$$

$$= 139.8 \text{ mg per day}$$

(b) Now the ranitidine comes as liquid, so this amount of medication must be expressed as milliliters.

15 mg/mL means that every 1 mL of the liquid contains 15 mg ranitidine

$$15 \text{ mg} \rightarrow 1 \text{ mL}$$
$$139.8 \text{ mg} \rightarrow u$$

$$U = \frac{1 \text{ mL}}{15 \text{ mg}} \times \frac{139.8 \text{ mg}}{1}$$

$$= 9.32 \text{ mL}$$

So the patient should take 9.32 mL per day.

Total authorized volume to be dispensed is for 30 days.

$$9.32 \text{ mL} \times 30 = 279.6 \text{ mL}.$$

(c) To calculate the amount of ranitidine (in milligrams) consumed in 30 days, we have two options

a) Multiply the daily milligrams consumed by 30 days. That is,

$$139.8 \text{ mg/day} \times 30 \text{ days}$$

$$= 4,194 \text{ mg}$$

or

b) Get the milligrams equivalent of the total volume dispensed. That is,

$$15 \text{ mL suspension} \rightarrow 1 \text{ mg ranitidine}$$
$$279.6 \text{ mL suspension} \rightarrow u$$

$$u = \frac{1 \text{ mg}}{15 \text{ mL}} \times \frac{279.6 \text{ mL}}{1}$$

$$= 4,194 \text{ mg}$$

Example 6.13

The usual initial dose of a particular drug is 150 mg/kg of body weight. How many milligrams should be administered to a patient weighing 154 pounds?

Solution

First, we convert the patient's weight from pound to kilogram because the dosage is expressed per kilogram.

$$2.2 \text{ pounds} \rightarrow 1 \text{ kg}$$
$$154 \text{ pounds} \rightarrow u$$
$$u = \frac{1 \text{ kg}}{2.2 \text{ pounds}} \times \frac{154 \text{ pounds}}{1}$$
$$= 70 \text{ kg}$$

Dosage calculations

$$1 \text{ kg body weight} \rightarrow 150 \text{ mg}$$
$$70 \text{ kg body weight} \rightarrow u$$
$$u = \frac{150 \text{ mg}}{1 \text{ kg body weight}} \times \frac{70 \text{ kg body weight}}{1}$$
$$= 10,500 \text{ mg}$$

Example 6.14

Consider the following prescription:

> Rx
>
> Amoxicillin 42 mg/kg/day in 3 divided doses.
>
> Dispense enough volume for 10 days.

Amoxicillin comes as 250 mg / 5 mL suspension when reconstituted. Patient weighs 44 pounds.

(a) What volume of the suspension in milliliters will make up the daily dose?
(b) What volume of the suspension in milliliters will make up a single dose?
(c) What volume of the suspension in milliliters must be dispensed to the patient enough for a ten-day regimen?

(d) Write out the instructions on the label.

(e) At the end of the ten days, what quantity of amoxicillin in grams would the patient have consumed?

Solution

(a) First, express the patient's weight as kilograms because the dosage is expressed per kg.

$$2.2 \text{ pounds} \rightarrow 1 \text{ kg}$$

$$44 \text{ pounds} \rightarrow u$$

$$u = \frac{1 \ kg}{2.2 \ pounds} \times \frac{44 \ pounds}{1}$$

$$= 20 \text{ kg}$$

$$1 \text{ kg body weight} \rightarrow 42 \text{ mg amoxicillin}$$

$$20 \text{ kg body weight} \rightarrow u$$

$$u = \frac{42 \ mg \ Amoxicillin}{1 \ kg \ body \ weight} \times \frac{20 \ kg \ body \ weight}{1}$$

$$= 840 \text{ mg amoxicillin per day}$$

So the patient takes a total of 840 mg of amoxicillin for the whole day.

Calculation of the volume that makes up a daily dose

$$250 \text{ mg amoxicillin} \rightarrow 5 \text{ mL suspension}$$

$$840 \text{ mg amoxicillin} \rightarrow u$$

$$u = \frac{5 \ mL \ suspension}{250 \ mg \ amoxicillin} \times \frac{840 \ mg \ amoxicillin}{1}$$

$$= 16.8 \text{ mL suspension per day}$$

(b) The physician was quick to add that the daily dose should be in three divided doses. Hence, we need to divide the daily dose into three equal parts to get each individual dose.

$$16.8 \text{ mL} \div 3 = 5.6 \text{ mL}$$

So a single dose in milliliters is 5.6 mL

(c) Volume to be dispensed

= daily volume consumed × number of days

= 16.8 mL × 10 = 168 mL

But because amoxicillin suspension comes in pack sizes of 75 mL, 100 mL, and 150 mL, it will be most economical to dispense one bottle of 75 mL and one bottle of 100 mL pack sizes, with instructions to discard the remainder after ten days of consumption.

(d) Instructions on the label

"Give 5.6 mL three times daily for 10 days,
then discard the remaining portion."

(e) This can be calculated from the daily milligrams consumed × number of days

= 840 mg/day × 10 days

= 8,400 mg

= 8.4 g

Or we can simply calculate the amount of amoxicillin contained in the total volume to be consumed by the patient.

Total volume to be consumed by patient is 168 mL.

5 mL suspension → 250 mg amoxicillin

168 mL suspension → u

$$u = \frac{250 \; mg \; amoxicillin}{5 \; mL \; suspension} \times \frac{168 \; mL \; suspension}{1}$$

= 8,400 mg

= 8.4 g

Chapter 6 Practice Questions

1. How many tablets of Tylenol will be dispensed to a patient with the following prescription?

   Tylenol Regular 325 mg

   Sig: i–ii Q8H PRN

       for 10 days

2. What is the daily dose for the following prescription?

   Tylenol #3

   Sig: i–ii po Q6–8H PRN

       M: 100

3. Consider this prescription:

   Metoprolol 25 mg po BID

   50 days

   How many tablets of 50 mg metoprolol should be dispensed to the patient for 50 days?

4. Consider the following prescription:

   Tylenol #4

   1–2 po Q4–6H PRN

   Supply 24 tablets

   a) What is the maximum single dose?
   b) What is the maximum daily dose?
   c) What duration will be assigned to the 24 tablets?

5. Consider the following prescription:

 Advil 600 mg

 1–2 tab Q6–8H PRN

$$\frac{1}{12}$$

a) What is the maximum single dose?
b) What is the maximum daily dose?
c) How many tablets should be dispensed for the entire duration ($\frac{1}{12}$) of the therapy?

6. Consider the following prescription

 Cefprozil suspension 125 mg / 5 mL

 Give 300 mg po TID

 Supply for 8 days

a) What is the single dose in milliliters?
b) What is the daily dose in milliliters?
c) How many milliliters will the patient consume at the end of therapy?
d) Write out the correct instructions on the label for the patient
e) If Cefprozil comes in standard pack sizes of 75 mL, 100 mL, and 150 mL, suggest the most economical way of dispensing different pack sizes to minimize waste and save cost.
f) How many milligrams of Cefprozil will the patient consume at the end of therapy?

7. The dosage of Cotridin syrup is 10 mL po TID. How long will 360 mL last for a patient if the medication is consumed as prescribed?

8. Consider the following prescription

   Tobradex ophth drops

   Sig: ii gtt OU BID

   M: 5 mL

   a) Interpret the sig
   b) How many drops will the patient instill into the eyes per day?
   c) How long will the 5 mL last the patient?

9. If 20 mL of a liquid medication contains fifty doses, how many drops will make up a dose? The dispensing dropper calibrates 20 drops per milliliter.

10. It takes 5 g of a cream to cover a patient's psoriasis in the elbow. If a physician prescribes the cream to be applied four times a day for ten days, what quantity of the cream should be dispensed?

11. A cold medication contains 30 mg of medication in one pint of the liquid. If the dosage of the cold medication is 1 tablespoon, how many milligrams of medication is contained in each dose?

12. Consider the following compounding formula:

    Robitussin 0.24 g

    Guaifenesin 1.2 g

    Simple syrup qs 100 mL

    Sig: one tbsp for wet cough

    How many milligrams of Robitussin and guaifenesin are contained in each tablespoon dose?

13. Dexamethasone injection solution contains 10 mg of active ingredient in each 4 mL of solution. If a medication order calls for 7.5 mg dexamethasone, how many milliliters should be administered?

14. In five days, 50 mL of a liquid medication is to be taken twice every day. How many teaspoonfuls should make up one dose?

15. Amoxicillin oral suspension 250 mg / 5 mL was prescribed 125 mg tid for ten days. If the available stock is 125 mg / 5 mL, consider the following questions:

    a) How many milliliters should be dispensed per dose?
    b) How many milliliters will form the daily dose?
    c) How many milliliters should be dispensed altogether to the patient for the entire duration of therapy?
    d) How many milligrams of amoxicillin will be consumed throughout the regimen?

16. The dose of a medication is 1.5 mg. How many teaspoons of the liquid medication containing 100 mcg/mL should be given to a patient to provide the 1.5 mg dosage?

17. A prescription calls for codeine sulfate 60 mg Q6–8h PRNP. The codeine tablet available in the pharmacy is labeled 15 mg per tablet.

    a) What is the single dose (number of tablets) using the 15 mg?
    b) What is the maximum daily dose (number of tablets) using the 15 mg?
    c) How many days will you assign as the approximate duration for 320 tablets?
    d) What will be the appropriate instruction on the label considering the availability of 15 mg tablets?

18. A physician orders the following:

> Metronidazole tabs 500 mg
>
> Sig: i PO TID UF
>
> > M: 10/7

> Metronidazole 500 mg capsules are not covered by the patient's insurance. The patient agrees to take metronidazole 250 mg strength, which is covered by insurance.

a) How many tablets of the 250 mg should be given per dose?
b) How many tablets should the patient consume per day?
c) How many tablets should be dispensed altogether for the entire regimen?

19. You receive the following prescription:

> Prednisolone 40 mg once daily
>
> Decrease by 5 mg Q week until done.

> If the available prednisolone is 5 mg per tablet, calculate the following:

a) How many tablets should be dispensed to the patient?
b) How long will it likely take to complete the regimen?

20. Due to a patient's palpitations, the physician orders bisoprolol 5 mg on even days and 7.5 mg on odd days. Only the 5 mg bisoprolol is available. Calculate how many tablets would be dispensed to the patient from the period of September 1 to September 30.

21. If the dosage of a solid oral medication is $\frac{1}{2}$ tablet on alternate days, how many tablets should be used to fill a forty-day order?

22. A physician orders the following:

        Valtrex 2 g po BID
           1/52

        The available Valtrex is 500 mg per tablet.

    (a) How many tablets should be given per dose?
    (b) How many tablets should form the daily dose?
    (c) How many tablets should be dispensed for the entire regimen?

23. Vagifem 10 mg was prescribed for a patient's menopausal symptoms. The instruction is to insert one tablet vaginally three times per week for three months. Approximately how many tablets should be dispensed to satisfy the duration?

24. You receive the following prescription:

        Cotridin expectorant liquid
        Sig: 5–10 mL Q6–8H PRN cough
           M: 200 mL

        The patient requested that you dispense just enough for two days. How many milliliters are you likely to dispense?

25. Calculate the authorized quantities of medication in the following prescriptions:

    (a) Colchicine 0.6 mg
         Sig: i–ii BID PRN 3/7

    (b) Tylenol Regular Strength
         Sig: i QID 10/7

(c) Flexeril 10 mg tablets

Sig: 20 mg po TID PRN

1/52

(d) Biaxin XL 500 mg

Sig: 1 gram po OD 2/52

(e) Codeine phosphate tablets 30mg

Sig: ss tablets tid 3/12

26. Calculate the number of days (duration) to be assigned to the following prescriptions.

(a) Tylenol #3

Sig: i tab Q8H PRN

M: 120 tablets

(b) Naproxen EC 375 mg

Sig: ii QID PRN

400 tablets

(c) Baclofen 10 mg

Sig: $\frac{1}{2}$ tablet TID

M: 150

(d) Clarithromycin tablet 500 mg

Sig: i po BID UF

M: 20

27. Calculate the authorized quantities of medication in the following prescriptions.

   (a) Tylenol #4
   Sig: i–ii TID PRN 8/7

   (b) Robaxasil C1/4
   Sig: ii po Q6–8H PRN
   1/12

   (c) Ranitidine liquid 15 mg/mL
   Sig: 112.5 mg po QHS 3/52

   (d) Amoxicillin 250 mg / 5 mL
   Sig: 400 mg TID UF 10/7

In question 28 to 32

Calculate the number of days (duration) to be assigned to the prescriptions as written.

28. Capsules amoxicillin 250 mg
   Sig: 500 mg po TID UF
   60 capsules

29. Zofran syrup 5 mg/mL
   Sig: 15 mg TID UD
   288 mL

30. Cotridin syrup
   Sig: 2 tbsp QHS
   M: 1 pint

31. Septrin suspension

      Sig: 1 tsp QID

          M: 200 mL

32. Lactulose syrup

      Sig: 2 tbsp BID

          M: 5 cups

In question 33 to 38

Calculate the quantity of medication to be dispensed to the patient according to the prescriptions written.

33. Tablets metoprolol 50 mg

      Sig: Take 25 mg BID 3/12

          (50 mg tabs available)

34. Flagyl capsules 500 mg

      Sig: i po TID for 10 days

          (Only 250 mg tablets available)

35. Tablets Fosamax 70 mg

      Sig: I Q week 3/12

36. Syrup morphine 5 mg/mL

      Sig: 5 mL EOD for 20 days

37. Tablet Norvasc 5 mg

   Sig: i QAM and 1.5 tablets QPM

       30 days

38. Capsules Losec 20 mg

   Sig: 2 capsules Q12H for 30 days.

39. A pediatric injection solution contains 200 mcg of the active ingredient per milliliters of the solution. What volume of the solution must be administered to provide a dose of 0.12 mg of the medication?

40. Mersyndol tablets

   Sig: ii tabs Q4–6H PRN for 15 days

   How many tablets should be dispensed to the patient?

41. How many milliliters of a pediatric suspension containing 40 mg of the active ingredient in each 8 mL should be used in filling a medication order calling for 25 mg three times per day for fifteen days?

42. Statex syrup 5 mg/mL

   Sig: 15 mg Q6H PRN

       300 mL

   What will be the duration of the therapy if medication is taken as prescribed?

43. If a compounded antihypertensive medication contains 0.10 g of amlodipine in every 3 mL of the suspension, how many milligrams of the amlodipine will be present in each tablespoon dose?

44. Keflex suspension 125 mg / 5 mL

    Sig: 750 mg po QID UF 2/52

    How many milliliters will the patient consume for two weeks, according to the prescription?

45. How many tablets of methotrexate will be dispensed in the following prescription?

    Rx

    Tab methotrexate (methotrexate sodium 2.5 mg per tablet)

    Sig: 20 mg PO Qwk

    　　3/12

46. A physician reduced the dosage of a hypothyroid patient from Synthroid 100 mcg once daily to a half tablet of 175 mcg every other day. What is the total reduction in levothyroxine (active ingredient in Synthroid) consumed in milligrams during a forty-five-day period?

47. Consider this prescription:

    Biaxin (Clarithromycin)15 mg/kg/day in divided doses Q12H for 10 days

    Patient weight is 22 pounds, and Biaxin is available as 125 mg / 5 mL suspension.

    (a) Calculate the daily dose for the child in milliliters.
    (b) Calculate the single dose for the child in milliliters.

(c) What amount of Biaxin suspension in milliliters should be consumed by the patient at the end of therapy?

(d) What amount of clarithromycin in gram should be consumed by patient at the end of the ten-day period?

(e) Write out the clear label instructions for the patient.

48. Consider the prescription below:

Dalacin C liquid 8–25 mg/kg/day in four divided doses.

Patient weighs 48 pounds, and Dalacin C is available in the pharmacy in a labeled strength of 75 mg / 5 mL.

(a) Calculate the daily dosage range in milligrams for the child.
(b) Calculate the daily dosage range in milliliters for the child.
(c) Calculate the single dosage range in milligrams for the child.
(d) Calculate the single dosage range in milliliters for the child.

49. Consider the prescription below:

Azithromycin 10 mg/kg/day as a single dose for day 1, followed by 5 mg/kg/day once daily for days 2 to 5.

Patient weighs 68 pounds, and azithromycin comes as 200 mg / 5 Ml suspension after proper reconstitution.

(a) What is the patient's single dose in milliliters for day 1?
(b) What is the patient's daily dose in milliliters for days 2 to 5?
(c) How many milliliters is the patient expected to consume for the entire duration of therapy?
(d) Design a suitable label instruction for the patient.

50. Consider the following prescription:

Zofran 0.9 mg/kg/dose every eight hours for ten days

Patient weighs 28 pounds, and Zofran liquid is available as 4 mg / 5 mL

(a) Calculate the single dose for the child in milliliters.
(b) Calculate the daily dose for the child in milliliters.
(c) What volume of the Zofran liquid will be dispensed to the patient?
(d) What amount of the active ingredient in g will be contained in the total authorized volume to be dispensed to the child?

★ Star Question ★

A prescription order calls for ceftriaxone 50 mg/kg for IM injection to a child whose weight is 39.6 pounds. The attending nurse injected 6 mL of a 200 mg/mL ceftriaxone suspension IM to the child. How many milligrams overdose of the ceftriaxone did the child receive?

Answers to Chapter 6
Practice Questions

1. 60 tablets
2. 8 tablets
3. 50 tablets
4. (a) 2 tablets
   (b) 12 tablets
   (c) 2 days
5. (a) 2 tablets
   (b) 8 tablets
   (c) 240 tablets
6. (a) 12 mL
   (b) 36 mL
   (c) 288 mL
   (d) Give 12 mL orally three times daily for eight days, then discard
      the remainder
   (e) 2 bottles of 150 mL pack size
   (f) 7,200 mg
7. 12 days
8. (a) Instill 2 drops into both eyes twice daily
   (b) 8 drops
   (c) approx. 12 days
9. 8 drops
10. 200 g
11. 0.9375 mg
12. 36 mg Robitussin
    180 mg guaifenesin
13. 3 mL
14. 1 tsp
15. (a) 5 mL
    (b) 15 mL
    (c) 150 mL
    (d) 3,750 mg
16. 3 tsp

17. (a) 4 tablets
    (b) 16 tablets
    (c) 20 days
    (d) Take 4 tablets (60 mg) every six to eight hours as needed for pain
18. (a) 2 tablets
    (b) 6 tablets
    (c) 60 tablets
19. (a) 252 tablets
    (b) 56 days
20. 37.5 tablets
21. 10 tablets
22. (a) 4 tablets
    (b) 8 tablets
    (c) 56 tablets
23. Approx. 38 tablets
24. 80 mL
25. (a) 12 tablets
    (b) 40 tablets
    (c) 42 tablets
    (d) 28 tablets
    (e) 135 tablets
26. (a) 40 days
    (b) 50 days
    (c) 100 days
    (d) 10 days
27. (a) 48 tablets
    (b) 240 tablets
    (c) 157.5 mL
    (d) 240 mL
28. 10 days
29. 32 days
30. 16 days
31. 10 days
32. 20 days
33. 90 tablets
34. 60 tablets

35. Approx. 13 tablets
36. 50 mL
37. 75 tablets
38. 120 capsules
39. 0.6 mL
40. 180 tablets
41. 225 mL
42. 25 days
43. 500 mL
44. 1,680 mL
45. Approx. 104 tablets
46. 2,531.25 mcg
47. (a) 6 mL
    (b) 3 mL
    (c) 60 mL
    (d) 1.5 g
    (e) Give 3 mL every twelve hours for ten days only
48. (a) 174.55 mg – 545.45 mg
    (b) 11.64 mL – 36.36 mL
    (c) 43.64 mg – 136.36 mg
    (d) 2.91 mL – 9.09 mL
49. (a) 7.73 mL
    (b) 3.86 mL
    (c) 23.17 mL
    (d) Give 7.73 mL as a single dose on day 1, then give 3.86 mL once daily for days 2 to 5 only as directed
50. (a) 4.8 mL
    (b) 14.3 mL
    (c) 143 mL
    (d) 0.1145 g

Solution to Star Question

The real dosage prescribed for the child can be calculated by following these steps.

Convert the child's weight from pound to kilograms because the dosage is per kg.

$$2.2 \text{ lb} \rightarrow 1 \text{ kg}$$

$$39.6 \text{ lb} \rightarrow u$$

$$u = \frac{1 \text{ kg}}{2.2 \text{ lb}} \times \frac{39.6 \text{ lb}}{1}$$

$$= 18 \text{ kg}$$

The child receives 50 mg per kg body weight, so the child's dosage should be

$$1 \text{ kg} \rightarrow 50 \text{ mg}$$

$$18 \text{ kg} \rightarrow u$$

$$u = \frac{50 \text{ mg}}{1 \text{ kg}} \times \frac{18 \text{ kg}}{1}$$

$$= 900 \text{ mg}$$

The nurse injected 6 mL of 200 mg/mL ceftriaxone. The actual milligrams injected by the nurse is:

$$1 \text{ mL} \rightarrow 200 \text{ mg}$$

$$6 \text{ mL} \rightarrow u$$

$$u = \frac{200 \text{ mg}}{1 \text{ mL}} \times \frac{6 \text{ mL}}{1}$$

$$= 1,200 \text{ mg}$$

The child was overdosed by:

$$1,200 \text{ mg} - 900 \text{ mg} = 300 \text{ mg}$$

CHAPTER 7

Calculations Surrounding Extemporaneous Preparations

Objectives

At the end of this chapter, students should be able to do the following:

- Apply proportion principles in the calculations involving different kinds of extemporaneous preparations.

Introduction

Every pharmacy professional will at one point or the other be confronted with the challenge of making some extemporaneous preparations for patients for one reason or another. Through the process of compounding, certain preparations are made in the pharmacy for the patient in order to satisfy both the physician requirements and specific patient needs. The Alberta College of Pharmacists (ACP), as well as other Canadian provincial pharmacy regulatory authorities, through their Standards for the Operations of Licensed Pharmacies, stipulates that each pharmacy must ensure that patients have access to compounding services. Thus, every licensed pharmacy in Canada must be capable of providing compounding services to the patients at least within limits of comfort and should be able to refer a patient to another pharmacy for compounding if the pharmacy is not able to prepare a prescribed compound for the patient.

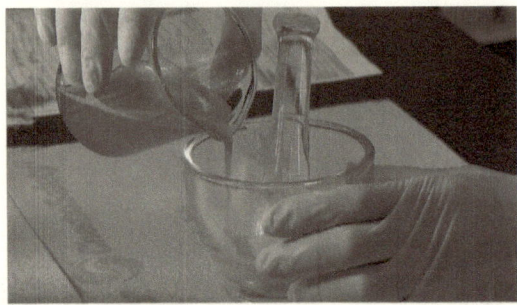

FIGURE7.1 *Pharmaceutical Compounding:* Through the process of extemporaneous preparations, health professionals are able to meet some specific patients' needs such as concentration, strength, consistency, flavor, taste and changes to a desired dosage form of medicinal formulations.

Compounding activities present themselves with various calculation challenges ranging from very simple math to a very complex calculation. Most of these calculations involve simple proportions. Background knowledge of compounding procedures as well as some compounding terms will be essential in compounding, but these are outside the scope of this book.

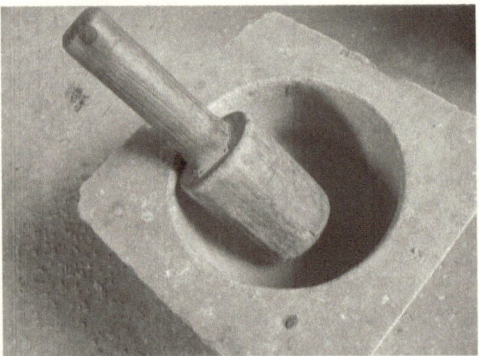

FIGURE 7.2 *Ancient Wooden Mortar and Pestle:* Pharmaceutical compounding is as old as pharmacy practice. The historic wooden mortar and pestle was probably used by the apothecaries for mixing and compounding of medicinal remedies.

The focus of this chapter will be on the calculations involved in the compounding of different types of pharmaceutical regimens in a community pharmacy. The following calculation examples will usher us into the world of calculations involving extemporaneous preparations.

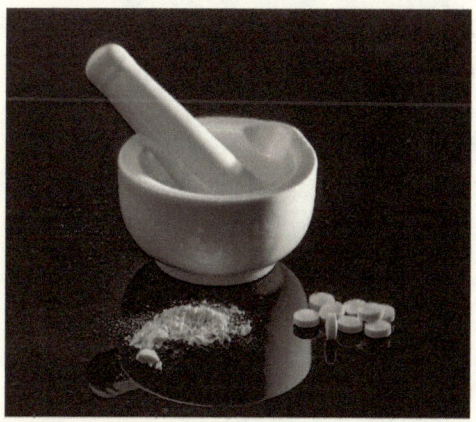

FIGURE 7.3 *The Ceramic Mortar and Pestle:* The Ceramic mortar and pestle remain a very powerful tool in pharmaceutical compounding for crushing, pulverizing, and mixing (trituration) of tablets, granules, crystals and other coarse solid particles to fine powder before incorporation of bases (or vehicles) to form creams, ointments, suspensions, pastes, et cetera.

Example 7.1

Consider the following prescription:

Rx

Diclofenac 8% in Diffusimax

Sig: AAA TID PRN

M: 250 g

(a) How many grams of diclofenac powder are needed to make the 250 g of the diclofenac gel?

(b) How many grams of Diffusimax will be needed in making the 250 g of the diclofenac gel?

Solution

Proper solution to this problem will start from accurate interpretation of the percentage of the diclofenac gel as prescribed.

An amount of 8% diclofenac in Diffusimax means that every 100 g of the diclofenac gel (the compound) must contain 8 g of the pure diclofenac powder.

Hence, we can say

$$100 \text{ g preparation} \rightarrow 8 \text{ g diclofenac}$$

$$250 \text{ g preparation} \rightarrow u$$

$$u = \frac{8 \text{ g } diclofenac}{100 \text{ g } preparation} \times \frac{250 \text{ g } preparation}{1}$$

$$= 20 \text{ g diclofenac powder}$$

So, to make 250 g of 8% diclofenac, in Diffusimax, I will need 20 g of the pure diclofenac powder.

(b) Realize that the compound is made by mixing pure diclofenac powder plus Diffusimax.

$$\text{diclofenac} + \text{Diffusimax} = \text{compound}$$

$$20 \text{ g diclofenac} + \text{Diffusimax} = 250 \text{ g compound}$$

$$\text{Diffusimax} = 250 \text{ g} - 20 \text{ g} = 230 \text{ g}$$

Therefore, to make 250 g of the compound, I simply need to blend together 20 g of pure diclofenac powder and 230 g of the Diffusimax. This will yield a homogenous mixture called 8% diclofenac gel.

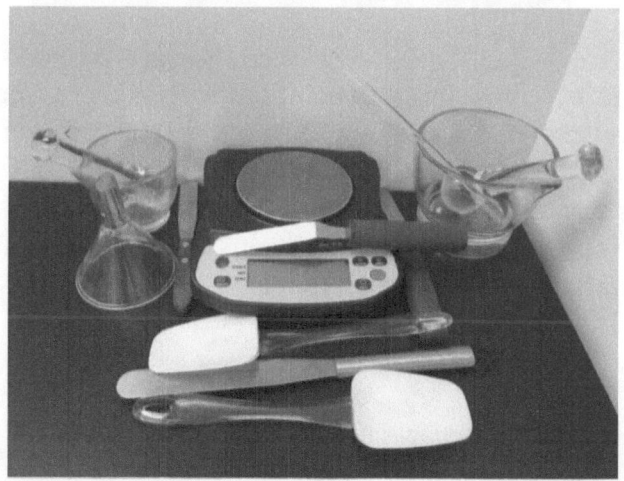

FIGURE 7.4 *Some Common Compounding Equipment:* Compounding in the pharmacy can be accomplished through the use of some simple compounding equipment as shown above such as: the mortar and pestle, the spatula, the weighing scale, the scraper, the stirring rod, the funnel, and so on.

Example 7.2

The following prescription was brought in by a patient:

Rx

Cyclobenzaprine 7% menthol 5% lidocaine 6% in PLO Gel

Sig: Apply to left knee QHS PRN

M: 300 g

(a) How many grams of cyclobenzaprine will be needed?
(b) How many grams of menthol will be needed?
(c) How many grams of lidocaine will be needed?
(d) How many grams of PLO Gel will be needed to make the 300 g of the compound?

Solution

(a) The cyclobenzaprine content of the final preparation is 7%, which means that every 100 g of the final preparation must contain only 7 g of cyclobenzaprine. In effect, this question is wondering, if 7 g of cyclobenzaprine must be in 100 g of the preparation, how many grams of cyclobenzaprine will be contained in 300 g of the preparation?

So we go,

$$100 \text{ g preparation} \rightarrow 7 \text{ g cyclobenzaprine}$$

$$300 \text{ g preparation} \rightarrow u$$

$$u = \frac{7 \text{ g cyclobenzaprine}}{100 \text{ g of preparation}} \times \frac{300 \text{ g of preparation}}{1}$$

$$= 21 \text{ g of cyclobenzaprine}$$

(b) The menthol content is 5%, which means that every 100 g of the preparation should contain 5 g of menthol. Similarly, using proportion, we can say

$$100 \text{ g preparation} \rightarrow 5 \text{ g menthol}$$

$$300 \text{ g preparation} \rightarrow u$$

$$u = \frac{5 \text{ g menthol}}{100 \text{ g of preparation}} \times \frac{300 \text{ g of preparation}}{1}$$

$$= 15 \text{ g of menthol}$$

(c) Similarly, calculating for lidocaine

$$100 \text{ g preparation} \rightarrow 6 \text{ g lidocaine}$$

$$300 \text{ g preparation} \rightarrow u$$

$$u = \frac{6 \text{ g lidocaine}}{100 \text{ g of preparation}} \times \frac{300 \text{ g of preparation}}{1}$$

$$= 18 \text{ g lidocaine}$$

(d) The compound is made by mixing all the component active ingredients with the base (PLO Gel) to make the topical preparation.

Now that we already know the amount of the active ingredients needed, the remaining weight of the compound will come from the base.

cyclobenzaprine + menthol + lidocaine + base = compound

$$21 \text{ g} + 15 \text{ g} + 18 \text{ g} + \text{PLO Gel} = 300 \text{ g}$$
$$\text{PLO Gel} = 300 \text{ g} - 21 \text{ g} - 15 \text{ g} - 18 \text{ g}$$
$$= 246 \text{ g}$$

Making this topical preparation will be as simple as crushing to very fine powder, the calculated quantities of cyclobenzaprine together with the menthol and lidocaine crystals in the mortar using the pestle, adding the base (PLO Gel), then triturating to a smooth and homogenous blend.

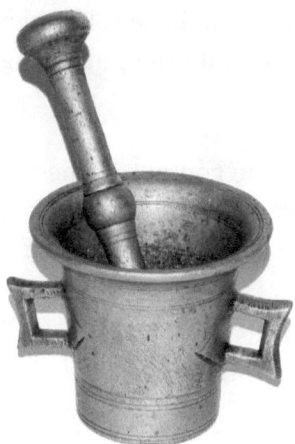

FIGURE 7.5 *The Old Brass Mortar and Pestle:* The Early century brass mortar and pestle used by the pioneers for extemporaneous preparation of pharmaceutical formulations

Example 7.3

A physician wants hydrocortisone powder to be blended into a commercially made Canesten cream for a baby with a very stubborn diaper rash. So the physician wrote the following prescription:

Rx

Hydrocortisone 2.5% in Canesten cream

Apply to diaper rash BID for 1 week

Make 150 gram

(a) What amount of hydrocortisone is needed for this compound?
(b) What amount of Canesten cream is needed for this compound?

Solution

In this type of compounding where some raw drug powder is incorporated into an already existing commercial (medicinal) preparation, the commercial preparation, for the purpose of calculations, is treated as the base (although we know it contains some active ingredients) while the pure drug powder is treated as the active ingredient.

(a) The hydrocortisone content of the final preparation will be 2.5%, which means that every 100 g of the preparation must contain 2.5 g of the hydrocortisone. So we can say

100 g preparation → 2.5 g hydrocortisone

150 g preparation → u

$$u = \frac{2.5 \text{ g hydrocortisone}}{100 \text{ g preparation}} \times \frac{150 \text{ g preparation}}{1}$$

= 3.75 g hydrocortisone powder

(b) Realize that the Canesten cream is already a preexisting formulated cream with its own DIN number. In this case, however, the Canesten cream is considered as a base (a sort of active base) because the hydrocortisone is meant to be incorporated into it. The Canesten cream will thus serve as the vehicle in which the hydrocortisone will be blended.

active ingredient + base = formulation

hydrocortisone + Canesten cream = formulation

3.75 g + Canesten cream = 150 g

Canesten cream = 150 g – 3.75 g

= 146.25 g of Canesten cream

Example 7.4

A physician ordered that a 1% clindamycin cream should be made. The physician further instructs that the base of the cream should be a 50:50 combination of nystatin cream and clotrimazole cream in the following prescription:

Rx

Clindamycin 1% in [nystatin:clotrimazole] (50:50)

Sig: Apply to rashes QHS PRN

Make 200 gram.

(a) What amount of clindamycin powder is needed?
(b) What amount of nystatin cream is needed?
(c) What amount of clotrimazole cream is needed?

Solution

The strength of the cream in terms of clindamycin content is 1%, which means that every 100 g of the final formulation must contain 1 g of clindamycin. So how many grams of clindamycin will be contained in 200 g of the formulation?

100 g formulation → 1 g clindamycin

200 g formulation → u

$$u = \frac{1\,g\,clindamycin}{100\,g\,formulation} \times \frac{200\,g\,formulation}{1}$$

$$= 2 \text{ g clindamycin powder}$$

If the active ingredient in the formulation of 200 g of a cream is 2 g, it means that the total amount of the base will be 200 g – 2 g = 198 g.

That is,

$$clindamycin + base = formulation$$

$$2 \text{ g clindamycin} + base = 200 \text{ g formulation}$$

$$base = 200 \text{ g} - 2 \text{ g}$$

$$= 198 \text{ g base}$$

But the base is a 50:50 combination of nystatin cream and clotrimazole cream. So the 198 g base represents a 50:50 blend of nystatin cream and clotrimazole cream. A proportion of 50:50 means both are present in equal proportion, which means that every 100 g of the base contains 50 g of nystatin cream and 50 g of clotrimazole cream. (See chapter 3 on ratios.)

(b) For nystatin cream

100 g base combination → 50 g nystatin

198 g base combination → u

$$u = \frac{50\,g\,nystatin}{100\,g\,base\,combination} \times \frac{198\,g\,base\,combination}{1}$$

$$= 99 \text{ g nystatin}$$

(c) For clotrimazole cream

100 g base combination → 50 g clotrimazole

198 g base combination → u

$$u = \frac{50\,g\,clotrimazole}{100\,g\,base\,combination} \times \frac{198\,g\,base\,combination}{1}$$

= 99 g clotrimazole cream

So to make the cream as prescribed, 2 g of clindamycin should be blended in a mixture of 99 g of nystatin cream and 99 g of clotrimazole cream, and the entire formulation will amount to 200 g.

That is to say,

2 g of clindamycin powder + 99 g of nystatin cream + 99 g of clotrimazole cream

= 200 g of formulation

Example 7.5

The following prescription was presented to the pharmacist:

Rx

Lamisil cream + Fucidin cream (3:2)

Sig: Apply to the affected area of the chest TID PRN

M: 450 grams

(a) What amount of Lamisil cream is needed to make the compound?
(b) What amount of Fucidin cream is needed to make the compound?

Solution

The solution to this problem lies in the proper understanding of the meaning of the combination ratio for the two ingredients in question (please review the chapter on ratios).

The combination ratio of 3:2 for Lamisil and Fucidin respectively means that every 5 g of the blended mixture must contain 3 g of Lamisil cream and 2 g of Fucidin cream.

5 g mixture → 3 g Lamisil cream + 2 g Fucidin cream

This equation defines the proportion and will be useful in the calculation of the amount of individual components of the formulation.

(a) For Lamisil cream

$$5 \text{ g mixture} \rightarrow 3 \text{ g Lamisil cream}$$
$$450 \text{ g mixture} \rightarrow u$$

$$u = \frac{3 \text{ g Lamisil cream}}{5 \text{ g mixture}} \times \frac{450 \text{ g mixture}}{1}$$

$$= 270 \text{ g Lamisil cream}$$

(b) For Fucidin cream

$$5 \text{ g mixture} \rightarrow 2 \text{ g Fucidin cream}$$
$$450 \text{ g mixture} \rightarrow u$$

$$u = \frac{2 \text{ g Fucidin}}{5 \text{ g mixture}} \times \frac{450 \text{ g mixture}}{1}$$

$$= 180 \text{ g Fucidin cream}$$

So 270 g Lamisil cream + 180 g Fucidin cream = 450 g of the compound.

Example 7.6

In order to manage very stubborn eczema due to the extreme dryness in the Northwest Territories of Northern Canada, a Yellowknife-based physician has developed his special formula, which is made by blending three topical preparations. The Rx is as follows:

Rx

CeraVe: Eucerin: Aquafor (6:8:5)

Sig: Apply to eczema areas TID

M: 380 grams

Calculate the amount of each ingredient needed to make 380 g of the special formula.

Solution

The solution to this problem begins with a proper grasp of the ratio formula.

$$6 + 8 + 5 = 19$$

The ratio means that

> every 19 g of the special bend must contain 6 g of CeraVe, 8 g of Eucerin, and 5 g of Aquaphor.

For CeraVe,

$$19 \text{ g blend} \rightarrow 6 \text{ g CeraVe}$$
$$380 \text{ g blend} \rightarrow u$$

$$u = \frac{6 \text{ g CeraVe}}{19 \text{ g blend}} \times \frac{380 \text{ g blend}}{1}$$

$$= 120 \text{ g of CeraVe}$$

For Eucerin,

$$19 \text{ g blend} \rightarrow 8 \text{ g Eucerin}$$
$$380 \text{ g blend} \rightarrow u$$

$$u = \frac{8 \text{ g Eucerin}}{19 \text{ g blend}} \times \frac{380 \text{ g blend}}{1}$$

$$= 160 \text{ g Eucerin}$$

For Aquaphor,

$$19 \text{ g blend} \rightarrow 5 \text{ g Aquaphor}$$
$$380 \text{ g blend} \rightarrow u$$

$$u = \frac{5 \text{ g Aquaphor}}{19 \text{ g blend}} \times \frac{380 \text{ g blend}}{1}$$

$$= 100 \text{ g Aquaphor}$$

The special formula must contain 120 g CeraVe, 160 g Eucerin, and 100 g Aquaphor. (120 + 160 + 100 = 380)

Example 7.7

The following liquid formulation was prescribed for an adult patient who had difficulty swallowing solid oral dosage forms:

> Rx
>
> Clindamycin 5% suspension in Ora-Blend
>
> Take 6 mL TID for 10 days.

What amount of clindamycin powder in grams is needed to make the entire suspension that will last for the ten days?

Solution

The first step in solving this is to determine the volume of the suspension that was actually prescribed. From the prescription above, the instruction is to take 6 mL of the compounded suspension three times daily for ten days.

This means the prescribed volume is

$$6 \text{ mL} \times 3 \times 10 = 180 \text{ mL}$$

Therefore, it is evident that 180 mL of the suspension must be dispensed to the patient in order to satisfy the demands of both dosage and duration of the prescription.

The second step is to determine what amount of the active ingredient will be needed to make the prescribed volume (180 mL)

The strength of 5% forms the basis for our proportional logic and will be useful for us in this calculation. A 5% suspension of clindamycin means that every 100 mL of the suspension must contain 5 g of the drug substance (clindamycin). Please see chapter 4 on the expressions of concentration.

So we can say

$$100 \text{ mL suspension} \rightarrow 5 \text{ g clindamycin}$$
$$180 \text{ mL suspension} \rightarrow u$$

$$u = \frac{5 \text{ } g \text{ } clindamycin}{100 \text{ } mL \text{ } suspension} \times \frac{180 \text{ } mL \text{ } suspension}{1}$$

$$= 9 \text{ g clindamycin powder}$$

Therefore, suspending 9 g of clindamycin in enough volume of Ora-Blend (quantity sufficient, qs)to make 180 mL of the suspension will produce a 5% clindamycin suspension.

Example 7.8

For the treatment of pediatric hypertension, the following prescription was issued to be compounded in the pharmacy for a child.

> Rx
>
> Amlodipine 0.05% suspension in simple syrup
>
> Sig: 3 mg PO QD 15/7

(a) Determine the volume of the suspension the pharmacy needs to make for the patient.
(b) What amount of amlodipine powder (active ingredient) is needed to make the suspension?
(c) If amlodipine is not available in the pharmacy as a pure powder but is available as tablets, each containing 5 mg of amlodipine, how many tablets will the pharmacist crush in order to obtain the required amount of active ingredient?
(d) Write out the correct instruction on the label for the patient.

Solution

(a) It should be noted that in this example, the dosage instruction is expressed in milligrams and not in milliliters (3 mg once daily for fifteen days).

The 3 mg represents a certain volume of the suspension. How many milliliters of the suspension will contain the 3 mg of amlodipine?

So let's first convert the 3 mg to volume. We can do this by taking our clue from the percentage of the suspension (0.05%).

A percentage of 0.05% means that every 100 mL of the suspension must contain 0.05 g of the active ingredient amlodipine. Remember that 3 mg is equivalent to 0.003 g (see chapter 2 on interconversion of units).

$$0.05 \text{ g amlodipine} \rightarrow 100 \text{ mL suspension}$$

$$0.003 \text{ g amlodipine} \rightarrow u$$

$$u = \frac{100 \text{ mL suspension}}{0.05 \text{ g amlodipine}} \times \frac{0.003 \text{ g amlodipine}}{1}$$

$$= 6 \text{ mL}$$

So 6 mL of the suspension will provide the needed 3 mg of the active ingredient, amlodipine.

The prescription can be interpreted as

$$6 \text{ mL (of the suspension) QD } 15/7$$

Total volume prescribed is

$$6 \text{ mL} \times 1 \times 15 = 90 \text{ mL}$$

(b) We can calculate the amount of the active ingredient in one of two ways.

Method 1: We can calculate that from the prescription itself.

$$3 \text{ mg} \times 1 \times 15 = 45 \text{ mg amlodipine}$$

Method 2: We can calculate the amount of amlodipine needed to make 90 mL of the suspension since we know that 0.05 g of amlodipine is contained in 100 mL of the suspension (0.05%).

100 mL suspension → 0.05 g amlodipine

90 mL suspension → u

$$u = \frac{0.05 \text{ g amlodipine}}{100 \text{ mL suspension}} \times \frac{90 \text{ mL suspension}}{1}$$

$$= 0.045 \text{ g amlodipine.}$$

This value in grams is equivalent to 45 mg.

(c) If we only have amlodipine tablets of 5 mg strength, a certain quantity of these tablets will yield 45 mg of the amlodipine. To calculate this, we take our logic from the fact that 1 tablet → 5 mg amlodipine.

Using our proportion and observing all the rules, we can say

5 mg amlodipine → 1 tab

45 mg amlodipine → u

$$u = \frac{1 \text{ tab}}{5 \text{ mg amlodipine}} \times \frac{45 \text{ mg amlodipine}}{1}$$

$$= 9 \text{ tabs}$$

Therefore, crushing nine tablets of the amlodipine tablets (5 mg per tablet) will yield 45 mg of the active ingredient amlodipine.

(d) To write out the label instruction for the patient, we need to be conscious of the fact that the instruction to the patient must be as clear as possible to avoid any form of ambiguity and to prevent medication error. In this case, advising the patient to take 3 mg of amlodipine from a suspension is not feasible because the final form of the product is a liquid measurable in milliliters.

So the instruction should read "Take 6 mL once daily for 15 days."

Example 7.9

Consider the following prescription:

Rx

Suspension Vasotec (enalapril) 7.5 mg / 5 mL in Ora-Sweet

Give 8 mL BID 10/7

(a) What volume of the suspension was prescribed to the patient?
(b) What amount of the active ingredient in milligrams is needed to make the suspension as prescribed?
(c) If Vasotec is not available in pure powder form in the pharmacy but is available as tablets, each containing 10 mg of the active ingredient (enalapril), how many tablets will be needed to make the suspension?

Solution

(a) The volume prescribed will be very clear from the prescription because the instruction is already in milliliters and not milligrams. An amount of 8 mL twice daily for ten days is

$$8 \text{ mL} \times 2 \times 10 = 160 \text{ mL}$$

(b) The amount of enalapril needed to make the suspension can be derived by finding the amount of enalapril that will be in 160 mL of the suspension if every 5 mL of the suspension must contain 7.5 mg enalapril (7.5 mg / 5 mL).

5 mL suspension ➔ 7.5 mg enalapril

160 mL suspension ➔ u

$$u = \frac{7.5\ mg\ enalapril}{5\ mL\ suspension} \times \frac{160\ mL\ suspension}{1}$$

= 240 mg enalapril

(c) Enalapril is available in the pharmacy as 10 mg tablets. That is to say that each tablet represents 10 mg of the active ingredients. So we can say

10 mg enalapril ➔ 1 tablet

240 mg enalapril ➔ u

$$u = \frac{1\ tablet}{10\ mg\ enalapril} \times \frac{240\ mg\ enalapril}{1}$$

= 24 tablets

Therefore, crushing 24 tablets of the (10 mg/tab) Vasotec and suspending it in enough Ora-Sweet to make a total volume of 160 mL will yield the enalapril suspension, whose strength will be 7.5 mg of enalapril per 5 mL of the suspension.

Example 7.10

In your pharmacy, you have a 12% diclofenac in Diffusimax already made. You also have 5% diclofenac in Diffusimax already made.

You receive the following prescription:

Rx

Diclofenac 10% in Diffusimax

Sig: AAA BID left knee PRN

M: 200 grams

Your desire is not to make a fresh batch of 10% diclofenac, but you want to mix both the 5% and the 12% together to make the 10%.

What quantities of the 5% and 12% must be mixed together to make the 200 grams of the 10%?

Solution

This can be solved comfortably using the alligation method. (Please see chapter 8 on alligation.)

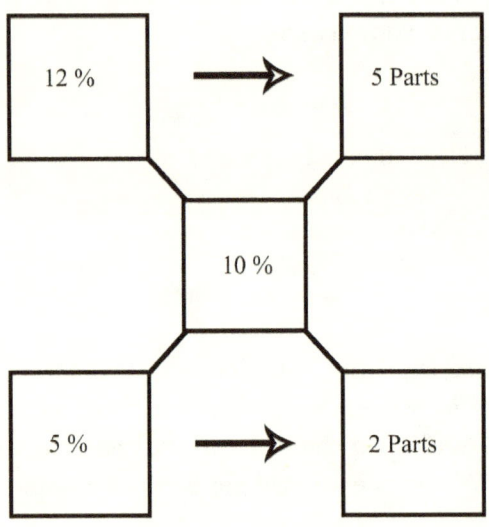

So the ratio of the 12% and 5% to be mixed to get the 10% is 5:2.

So 7 g of the mixture (10%) must contain 5 g of 12% and 2 gram of 5%

Calculating for 12%

$$7 \text{ g mixture (10\%)} \rightarrow 5 \text{ g (12\%)}$$
$$200 \text{ g mixture (10\%)} \rightarrow u$$

$$u = \frac{5 \text{ g (12\%)}}{7 \text{ g mixture (10\%)}} \times \frac{200 \text{ g mixture (10\%)}}{1}$$

$$= 142.86 \text{ g of 12\%}$$

Calculating for 5%

$$7 \text{ g mixture } (10\%) \rightarrow 2 \text{ g } (5\%)$$

$$200 \text{ g mixture } (10\%) \rightarrow u$$

$$u = \frac{2 \text{ g } (5\%)}{7 \text{ g mixture } (10\%)} \times \frac{200 \text{ g mixture } (10\%)}{1}$$

$$= 57.14 \text{ g of } 5\%$$

$$142.86 \text{ g } (12\%) + 57.14 \text{ g } (5\%) = 200 \text{ g of } 10\%$$

Example 7.11

A pharmacist crushed 80 tablets of 10 mg domperidone tablets in mortar with pestle. The pharmacist mixed the powder in enough Ora-Blend syrup to make 160 mL of domperidone suspension. What is the percentage strength of the resulting suspension made?

Solution

80 tablets of domperidone 10 mg tablets will yield

$$80 \times 10 = 800 \text{ mg of domperidone (active ingredient)}$$

Literally, it implies that 800 mg of domperidone is suspended in enough vehicle to make 160 mL.

Then, if 800 mg (0.8 g) of domperidone is contained in 160 mL of the suspension, how many grams will be contained in 100 mL of the suspension? The answer will define the percentage.

$$160 \text{ mL suspension} \rightarrow 0.8 \text{ g domperidone}$$

$$100 \text{ mL suspension} \rightarrow u$$

$$u = \frac{0.8 \text{ g domperidone}}{160 \text{ mL suspension}} \times \frac{100 \text{ mL suspension}}{1}$$

$$= 0.5 \text{ g domperidone in } 100 \text{ mL suspension}$$

If 0.5 gram of an active ingredient is contained in
100 mL of a suspension, the percentage is 0.5

Example 7.12

The contents of 20 capsules of amoxicillin 500 mg/cap were used to make 200 mL of amoxicillin suspension in Ora-Blend vehicle. What is the resultant concentration of the suspension in terms of mg/5 mL?

Solution

20 capsules of amoxicillin 500 mg cap will yield

$$20 \times 500 = 10,000 \text{ mg}$$

So if this amount of active ingredient is used to make 200 mL of the suspension, we can say the 200 mL of the suspension contains 10,000 mg of amoxicillin. Then how much of the amoxicillin (in milligrams) will be in 5 mL of the suspension? This is what the question seeks to know.

200 mL suspension → 10,000 mg amoxicillin

5 mL suspension → u

$$u = \frac{10,000 \ mg \ amoxicillin}{200 \ mL \ suspension} \times \frac{5 \ mL \ suspension}{1}$$

= 250 mg of amoxicillin in 5 mL of the suspension

= 250 mg / 5mL

Example 7.13

A pharmacy technician compounded some diclofenac ointment by mixing 10 g of diclofenac powder with 150 g of Diffusimax base. What is the percentage concentration of the diclofenac ointment compounded by the pharmacy technician?

Solution

When 10 g of diclofenac powder is mixed with 150 g of Diffusimax, the result is 160 g of the diclofenac ointment.

10 g diclofenac + 150 g Diffusimax = 160 g of diclofenac ointment.

So we can say that 10 g of diclofenac powder is contained in 160 g of the formulation (ointment). So how many grams of the diclofenac will be contained in 100 g of the formulation? The answer will represent the percentage concentration.

$$160 \text{ g formulation} \rightarrow 10 \text{ g diclofenac}$$
$$100 \text{ g formulation} \rightarrow u$$
$$u = \frac{10 \text{ g } diclofenac}{160 \text{ g } formulation} \times \frac{100 \text{ g } formulation}{1}$$

= 6.25 g of diclofenac in 100 g of the formulation, which means 6.25%

Example 7.14

A pharmacy technician has the intention of making 400 grams of 40% menthol ointment using menthol crystals (active ingredient) and Aquaphor as the neutral base. She later discovered she had only 150 grams of the Aquaphor and enough menthol. What is the maximum amount of the 40% menthol ointment she can make with the limited amount of the Aquaphor?

Solution

To make 200 grams of 40% menthol, the technician needs to mix

80 g of menthol + 120 g of Aquaphor = 200 g of the formulation

(or simply: 40 g menthol +60 g Aquaphor
= 100 g formulation i.e =40%)

271

Focusing on the Aquaphor and the formulation, it is clear that 120 grams of Aquaphor can make 200 grams of the formulation. This question wants to know how many grams of the formulation the 150 grams of available Aquaphor can make.

$$120 \text{ g Aquaphor} \rightarrow 200 \text{ g formulation}$$

$$150 \text{ g Aquaphor} \rightarrow u$$

$$u = \frac{200 \text{ } g \text{ } formulation}{120 \text{ } g \text{ } Aquaphor} \times \frac{150 \text{ } g \text{ } Aquaphor}{1}$$

$$= 250 \text{ g of the formulation}$$

Example 7.15

A pharmacist mixed 63 grams of Lamisil cream and 36 grams of Elocom cream on the ointment slab to form a homogeneous blend of Lamisil–Elocom mixture. What is the ratio of Lamisil to Elocom in the resultant mixture?

Solution

The mixture is as follows:

Lamisil : Elocom

63 g : 36 g

Dividing both sides by their common factor, 9, we will arrive at

Lamisil : Elocom

7 : 4

So the ratio of the mixture of Lamisil and Elocom is 7:4.

Chapter 7 Practice Questions

1. Consider the following prescription:

   Rx

   Hydrocortisone 2% ointment in Vaseline

   Sig: AAA TID PRN

       M: 150 grams

   Calculate

   (a) The amount of hydrocortisone in grams needed to make the compound
   (b) The amount of Vaseline in grams needed to make the compound.

2. Consider the following prescription:

   Rx

   Omeprazole (Losec) suspension 5 mg/mL in Ora-Blend

       Sig: Take 10 mg PO BID for 10 days

   Calculate the amount of omeprazole powder needed to make the authorized volume of the suspension.

3. A pharmacy technician crushed 15 grams of urea crystals to a very fine powder and blended it with 135 grams of PLO gel to make a topical urea gel. What is the percentage strength of the urea in the gel prepared?

4. You receive the following prescription:

    Rx

    Diclofenac 8%, menthol 5%, lidocaine 4% in Diffusimax

    Sig: AAA TID PRN UD

    Make 300 grams

    (a) What amount of diclofenac powder is needed to make the 300 grams of compound?
    (b) What amount of menthol crystal is needed to make the 300 grams of compound?
    (c) What amount of lidocaine powder is needed to make the 300 grams of compound?
    (d) What amount of Diffusimax is needed to make the 300 grams of compound?

5. Consider the following prescription for pediatric hypertension:

    Rx

    Enalapril suspension 0.1% in Ora-Sweet

    Sig: Take 5 mL BID for 15 days

    Calculate the amount of enalapril powder in grams needed to make the suspension that will last for fifteen days, according to the prescription.

6. Consider the following prescription:

    Rx

    Domperidone suspension 0.1% in simple syrup

    Sig: Take 10 mg QID for 10 days

    (a) How many milliliters of the suspension will the patient receive per unit dose according to the prescription?

(b) How many milliliters of the suspension will the patient receive per day according to the prescription?

(c) What amount of the active ingredient powder in milligrams will be needed to make the suspension as prescribed?

(d) If domperidone is not available as pure powder in the pharmacy but is only available as tablets, each containing 10 mg of domperidone, calculate the quantity of the tablets that need to be crushed in making the suspension.

7. You have available in the pharmacy 5% diclofenac gel and 8% diclofenac gel. You receive the following prescription:

> Rx
>
> Diclofenac gel 6%
>
> Apply as directed to affected areas
>
> Make 200 grams

What amount of diclofenac gel 5% and 8% will be needed to make the desired 200 grams of 6% diclofenac gel?

8. Approximately 50 amoxicillin capsules (500 mg/cap) were opened and the contents blended with enough simple syrup to make 80 mL suspension. How many milligrams of amoxicillin will be contained in each 10 mL of the suspension?

9. A pharmacy assistant was instructed to make 200 mL of 0.4% dexamethasone suspension in Ora-Sweet. Upon checking the stock, the pharmacy assistant discovered that only fifty tablets of 4 mg dexamethasone were available in stock and enough Ora-Sweet vehicle. What is the maximum volume of the suspension the pharmacy assistant can make using the available tablets?

10. A pharmacist has 8 mL of 50% dextrose solution. In order to dilute the solution, the pharmacist poured distilled water into the 8 mL to make the volume 100 mL. What is the new percentage strength of the diluted dextrose solution?

11. Consider the following physician order:

    Rx

    Diclofenac 8% in Diffusimax

    Apply to right elbow BID PRN

    　　M: 200 grams

    If the patient only needed 120 grams to be dispensed, calculate the following:

    (a) The amount of diclofenac powder (in grams) needed to make 120 grams of the compound.
    (b) The amount of Diffusimax (in grams) needed to make 120 grams of the compound.

12. Exactly 20 grams of menthol crystal were crushed to fine powder with mortar and pestle, and the powder was triturated with 140 grams of Eucerin as the base. What is the percentage strength of the menthol in the final compound formed?

13. You receive the following prescription:

    Rx

    Domperidone suspension 0.05% in Ora-Blend

    Sig: Give 7.5 mg PO QID AC for 10 days.

    Calculate the amount of domperidone powder needed to make ten days' supply of the suspension as prescribed.

14. Consider the following prescription:

    Rx

    Gabapentin 5%, lidocaine 4%, diclofenac 6% in Dermabase

    Sig: Apply as directed to affected areas

    M: 250 grams

    (a) What amount of gabapentin powder is needed to make 250 grams of the compound?
    (b) What amount of lidocaine powder is needed to make 250 grams of the compound?
    (c) What amount of diclofenac powder is needed to make 250 grams of the compound?
    (d) What amount of Dermabase is needed to make 250 grams of the compound?

15. You receive the following prescription:

    Rx

    Domperidone suspension 0.05% in simple syrup

    Sig: Take 20 mL AC breakfast 10/7

    Calculate the amount of domperidone powder needed to make the entire prescribed volume of the prescription.

16. You received an order from the physician instructing you to mix 160 grams of Fucidin cream and 280 grams of Fucidin ointment to make a homogenous blend of Fucidin cream/ointment. What is the ratio of Fucidin cream:Fucidin ointment in the blend?

17. You desire to make 500 grams of 10% urea ointment. You already have 5% urea ointment and 20% urea ointment in stock. What quantities of the 5% and 20% will need to be mixed to achieve your objective?

18. Approximately 40 tablets of enalapril 10 mg were crushed and suspended in enough Ora-Sweet to make a 120 mL suspension. What is the percentage strength of the resulting suspension?

19. A pharmacy technician was instructed to make 200 mL of domperidone suspension in simple syrup such that every 5 mL of the suspension must contain 10 mg of domperidone. The technician discovered he has only 20 tablets of domperidone (10 mg/tab) and enough simple syrup. What is the maximum volume of the suspension the pharmacy technician can make using the available number of 10 mg tablets?

20. A physician ordered the following:

   Rx

   Clindamycin cream 4% in Glaxal Base

   Sig: Apply externally to infected area TID

   M: 300 grams

   Calculate the following:

   (a) The amount of clindamycin powder in grams needed to make the compound
   (b) The amount of Glaxal Base in grams needed to make the compound

21. Approximately 80 grams of salicylic acid were crushed to fine powder and blended with 160 grams of petroleum jelly to make a topical salicylic acid ointment. What is the percentage concentration of salicylic acid in the resulting topical ointment prepared?

22. Consider the following prescription:

Rx

Clindamycin suspension 1.5% in Ora-Blend liquid

     Sig: Take 150 mg PO TID 10/7

(a) How many milliliters of the suspension will the patient receive per unit dose according to the prescription?
(b) How many milliliters of the suspension will the patient receive per day according to the prescription?
(c) What amount of the active ingredient (clindamycin) is needed to make the suspension as prescribed?
(d) If clindamycin is not available as pure powder in the pharmacy but only available as capsules, each containing 300 mg of clindamycin, calculate the number of the clindamycin capsules that will be emptied and whose contents will be crushed and used in making the suspension.

23. Consider the following prescription:

Rx

Esomeprazole suspension 10 mg / 3 mL

     Sig: Take 12 mL PO QD for 10 days.

Calculate the amount of esomeprazole powder in grams that will be needed to make the entire prescribed volume of the prescription.

24. The following is a prescription of a special emollient blend used in the treatment of eczema due to dryness.

Rx

Vaseline:Eucerin (4:5)

Sig: Apply to eczema area TID PRN

   Make 180 grams

(a) What amount of Vaseline will be needed to make 180 grams of the formula?
(b) What amount of Eucerin will be needed to make 180 gram of the formula?

25. Consider the following prescription for oral clindamycin suspension:

Rx

Clindamycin suspension 3% in Ora-Blend SF

   Sig: Give 5 mL TID for 10 days

Calculate the amount of clindamycin powder needed to make the entire authorized volume of the prescription.

26. Consider the following prescription:

Rx

Lamisil suspension 2.5% in Cherry syrup

   Sig: Give 250 mg PO BID for 20 days

(a) How many milliliters of the suspension will the patient receive per unit dose according to the prescription?
(b) How many milliliters of the suspension will the patient receive per day according to the prescription?
(c) What amount of the active ingredient is needed to make the suspension as prescribed?

(d) If Lamisil is not available as pure powder in the pharmacy but only available as tablets, each containing 250 mg of terbinafine, calculate the quantity of the tablets that need to be crushed in making the suspension.

27. A physician ordered 100 grams of 8% diclofenac ointment. Available in the pharmacy are two strengths of diclofenac ointment: 12% and 5%. What quantities of the available strengths will be mixed to make the prescribed quantity of the 8%?

28. Approximately 50 grams of dextrose were dissolved in enough distilled water to make 400 mL of dextrose solution.

    (a) What is the percentage strength of the dextrose solution?
    (b) How many grams of dextrose will be contained in each 10 mL of the prepared dextrose solution?

29. To make a special-tasting vehicle for oral suspension, a pharmacist added 40 mL of Ora-Sweet to a certain amount of simple syrup to make 110 mL of Ora-Sweet / simple syrup blend. What is the ratio of Ora-Sweet : simple syrup in the mixture?

30. Consider the following instruction:

    Clindamycin suspension 6% in Ora-Blend

    Make enough suspension with the
    available clindamycin powder.

    If the available clindamycin powder is 1.8 grams, what is the volume of the suspension that can be made?

31. Consider the compound based on the following prescription:

Rx

Gabapentin 12% ointment in Aquaphor

Sig: Apply to neuropathic feet TID

M: 250 grams

Calculate the following:

(a) The amount of gabapentin powder in grams needed to make the compound
(b) The amount of Aquaphor in grams needed to make the compound

32. Consider the following prescription:

Rx

Elocom cream : Canesten cream (5:7)

Sig: Apply to affected area BID UD

M: 120 grams

If only one tube of Elocom cream (× 30 grams) is available, what is the maximum amount of the mixture that can be made with the available Elocom cream?

33. A pharmacist mixed 3 grams of hydrocortisone powder with 122 grams of Dermabase to make a topical hydrocortisone preparation. What is the percentage strength of the resulting preparation made?

34. In order to treat a child's very stubborn diaper rash, the physician ordered the following:

Canesten cream: nystatin cream (3:2)

Sig: Apply BID to diaper rash then coat with Zincofax

M: 200 grams

Calculate the following:

(a) The amount of Canesten cream (in grams) needed to make the compound
(b) The amount of nystatin cream (in grams) needed to make the compound

35. To treat a child's fungal toe infection, the physician ordered the following prescription:

Rx

Lamisil suspension 3% in cherry syrup

Sig: Give 150 mg once daily for 20 days

× 5 Rpt

Calculate the amount of Lamisil powder (in grams) needed to make a twenty-day supply of the suspension.

36. The following is a prescription for an adult hypertensive patient with cancer of the esophagus who had difficulty swallowing pills:

Rx

Metoprolol suspension 10 mg / 5 mL

Sig: Take 25 mg PO BID for 10 days.

Calculate the amount of metoprolol powder needed to make the suspension.

37. You received the following prescription for the treatment of pediatric croup.

Rx

Dexamethasone suspension 2 mg/mL in Ora-Blend

    Sig: Give 8 mL Po QHS for 10 days

(a) How many milligrams of dexamethasone is prescribed per unit dose?
(b) What volume of the suspension will be dispensed to the patient to last for the ten days as prescribed?
(c) If dexamethasone is not available as pure powder in the pharmacy but is only available as tablets, each containing 4 mg of dexamethasone, how many tablets will be crushed in making the suspension as prescribed?

38. You are required to prepare 4 ounces of 12% potassium chloride solution using 20% potassium chloride solution and 8% potassium chloride solution. What volumes (in milliliters) of the 12% and the 8% will be needed to make the 4 ounces of your desired strength?

39. A pharmacy technician has the intention of making 300 grams of 8% diclofenac ointment in Vaseline. She eventually discovered that she has only 200 grams of Vaseline available in the pharmacy and enough diclofenac powder. What is the maximum amount of the ointment she can make with the available Vaseline?

40. A physician ordered that Ketoderm cream and Hyderm cream be mixed in the ratio of 3:2. The quantity ordered was 400 grams. What is the amount of Ketoderm cream and Hyderm cream that must be mixed in order to satisfy the ratio and the prescribed quantity?

41. You receive the following antihypertensive prescription from a patient who requested a liquid oral formulation.

Rx

Amlodipine suspension 7.5 mg / 5 mL in Ora-Sweet SF

Sig: Take 8 mL PO once daily 10/7

(a) How many milligrams of amlodipine will the patient receive per unit dose according to the prescription?
(b) How many milliliters of the suspension will the patient receive for ten days according to the prescription?
(c) What amount of the active ingredient is needed to make the suspension as prescribed?
(d) If amlodipine is not available as pure powder in the pharmacy but only available as tablets, each containing 5 mg of amlodipine, calculate the quantity of the tablets that need to be crushed in making the suspension.

42. A homogeneous blend of cream was made by mixing 200 grams of nystatin cream and 160 grams of Hyderm. What is the ratio of nystatin: Hyderm in the final blend?

43. A pharmacist wants to prepare 300 mL of 20 mg / 5 mL enalapril suspension in Ora-Blend. Upon checking her stock, she discovered that she has enough Ora-Blend vehicle but only eighty tablets (of 10 mg/tab) enalapril. What is the maximum volume of the enalapril suspension she can make with the available 10 mg tablets?

44. A physician wants to combine three topical agents to treat a chronic pediatric diaper rash, so he ordered the following:

Rx

Clotrimazole cream : Hyderm cream : Nyaderm cream (4:3:5)

Sig: Apply QHS to diaper rash

M: 360 grams

In order to make 360 grams of this special combination, calculate the following:

(a) The amount of clotrimazole cream needed
(b) The amount of Hyderm cream needed
(c) The amount of nystatin cream needed

45. You received the following prescription to be made in the pharmacy:

Rx

Amlodipine suspension 0.15% in Ora-Blend

Sig: Give 7.5 mg once daily for 20 days.

Calculate the amount of amlodipine powder needed to make enough of the suspension that will last for twenty days.

46. Consider the following prescription:

Rx

Enalapril 0.1% suspension in Ora-Blend

Sig: Take 5 mL PO BID for 10 days

(a) How many milligrams will the patient receive per unit dose according to the prescription?
(b) How many milligrams of enalapril will the patient receive per day according to the prescription?
(c) If enalapril is not available as pure powder in the pharmacy but only available as tablets, each containing 10 mg of enalapril, calculate the quantity of tablets that need to be crushed in making the suspension.

47. The following muscle relaxant was prescribed for a patient with back pain who preferred liquid oral dosage form:

   Rx

   Cyclobenzaprine (Flexeril) suspension
   10 mg / 3 mL in simple syrup

   Sig: Take 6 mL PO QHS PRN

       M: 120 mL

   (a) How many milligrams of cyclobenzaprine will the patient receive per unit dose according to the prescription?
   (b) How many milligrams of the cyclobenzaprine will the patient receive per day according to the prescription?
   (c) What amount of the active ingredient is needed to make the suspension as prescribed?
   (d) If cyclobenzaprine is not available as pure powder in the pharmacy but only available as tablets, each containing 10 mg of cyclobenzaprine, calculate the quantity of tablets that need to be crushed in making the suspension.

48. Twenty tablets of Plendil 10 mg tablets was crushed and suspended in enough Ora-Blend to make 120 mL of Plendil suspension. How many milligrams of Plendil will be contained in every 5 mL of the final suspension?

49. For the following prescription:

   Rx

   Felodipine suspension 0.1% in cherry syrup

       Sig: Give 5 mg once daily 2/52

   Calculate the amount of felodipine powder (in grams) needed to make the suspension that will last for two weeks.

---

50. A patient complained to the physician that he does not like using topical medications in ointment base. The physician, however, does not want to prescribe a cream-based topical application to the patient. The physician therefore decided to prescribe a blend of ointment and cream together in the following prescription:

> Rx
>
> Fucidin cream : Fucidin ointment (5:3)
>
> Sig: Apply to skin lesions TID UD
>
> M: 240 grams

(a) Calculate the amount of Fucidin cream needed to make 240 grams of the blend
(b) Calculate the amount of Fucidin ointment needed to make 240 grams of the blend.

★ Star Question ★

A pharmacy assistant wants to make 500 grams of 10% diclofenac ointment with the only available full bottle of diclofenac powder (1 full bottle = 50 grams) and enough PLO Gel. During the compounding, the assistant lost 8 grams of the powder due to a spill but went ahead to use the remaining 42 grams of the diclofenac powder. In order to achieve the original target of making 500 grams of the preparation, the assistant used the PLO Gel to make up for the 8 grams. What is the percentage strength of the diclofenac that was eventually made?

Answers to Chapter 7 Practice Questions

1. (a) 3 g hydrocortisone powder
   (b) 147 g Vaseline
2. 200 mg omeprazole powder
3. 10%
4. (a) 24 g diclofenac powder
   (b) 15 g menthol crystal
   (c) 12 g lidocaine
   (d) 249 g Diffusimax
5. 0.15 g enalapril powder
6. (a) 10 mL
   (b) 40 mL
   (c) 400 mg
   (d) 40 tablets
7. 66.667 g of 8%
   133.333 g of 5%
8. 3,125 mg
9. 50 mL
10. 4%
11. (a) 9.6 g diclofenac powder
    (b) 110.4 g Diffusimax
12. 12.5%
13. 300 mg
14. (a) 12.5 g gabapentin powder
    (b) 10 g lidocaine
    (c) 15 g diclofenac
    (d) 212.5 g Dermabase
15. 100 mg domperidone powder
16. 4:7 (Fucidin cream : Fucidin ointment)
17. 333.333 g of 5%
    166.667 g of 20%
18. 0.333%
19. 100 mL

20. (a) 12 g clindamycin
    (b) 288 g Glaxal Base
21. 33.33%
22. (a) 10 mL
    (b) 30 mL
    (c) 4,500 mg
    (d) 15 capsules
23. 0.4 g
24. (a) 80 g Vaseline
    (b) 100 g Eucerin
25. 4,500 mg
26. (a) 10 mL
    (b) 20 mL
    (c) 10 g
    (d) 40 tablets
27. 42.857 g of 12%
    57.143% of 5%
28. (a) 12.5%
    (b) 1.25 g dextrose
29. 4:7 (Ora-Sweet : simple syrup)
30. 30 mL
31. (a) 30 g gabapentin powder
    (b) 220 g Aquaphor
32. 72 g
33. 2.4%
34. (a) 120 g Canesten cream
    (b) 80 g nystatin cream
35. 3 g
36. 500 mg
37. (a) 16 mg dexamethasone
    (b) 80 mL suspension
    (c) 40 tablets
38. 80 mL of 8%
    40 mL of 20%
39. 217.39 g ointment
40. 240 g Ketoderm cream
    160 g Hyderm cream

41. (a) 12 mg
    (b) 80 mL
    (c) 120 mg
    (d) 24 tablets
42. 5:4 (Nystatin: Hyderm)
43. 200 mL
44. (a) 120 g clotrimazole cream
    (b) 90 g Hyderm cream
    (c) 150 g nystatin cream
45. 150 mg amlodipine powder
46. (a) 5 mg
    (b) 10 mg
    (c) 10 tablets
47. (a) 20 mg
    (b) 20 mg
    (c) 400 mg
    (d) 40 tablets
48. 8.33 mg
49. 0.07 g
50. (a) 150 g Fucidin cream
    (b) 90 g Fucidin ointment

Solution to Star Question

From the question, the technician eventually used

42 g of the diclofenac powder

458 g of the neutral base, PLO Gel

Total quantity of the formulation made is

42 g + 458 g = 500 g of diclofenac gel in PLO

So we can say that 42 grams of diclofenac powder is contained in 500 grams of the gel formulation. The percentage strength will be the quantity of diclofenac powder (in grams) that will be contained in 100 grams of the gel formulation. So we go

500 g gel formulation → 42 g diclofenac powder

100 g gel formulation → u

$$u = \frac{42 \ g \ diclofenac \ powder}{500 \ g \ gel \ formulation} \times \frac{100 \ g \ gel \ formulation}{1}$$

= 8.4 g diclofenac powder

So the formulation now contains 8.4 grams of diclofenac in every 100 grams of the formulation. This means 8.4 percent.

CHAPTER 8

Alligation Calculations

Objectives

At the end of this chapter, students should be able to do the following:

- Demonstrate understanding of the concept of alligation
- Outline the rules governing the alligation calculations
- Apply the alligation rules in basic alligation calculations

Introduction

Alligation is a mathematical method of solving calculations involving mixing of some compounds or some solution of different strengths (concentrations). Alligation seeks to calculate the different proportions of two given strengths of a compound that will yield a desired concentration of a specified quantity of the mixture.

When two different strengths of a given compound or solution are mixed together, the strength of the final mixture must lie between the strength of the weaker component and that of the stronger component.

For example, if 5% diclofenac in Diffusimax is mixed with 8% diclofenac in Diffusimax, the strength of the final mixture will lie somewhere between 5% and 8%. The relative amounts of the two components will determine if the final strength of the mixture will tend towards the weaker or the stronger component. If the mixture has more of 5%, the strength of the mixture will lie close to 5%, and if the mixture has more of 8%, the strength of the mixture will be closer to 8%.

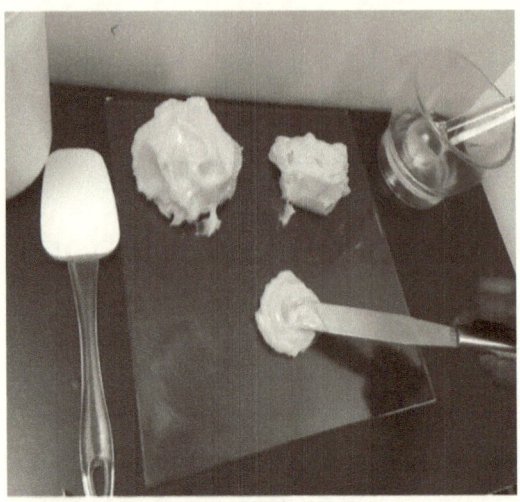

FIGURE 8.1 *Alligation:* Through alligation process, different strengths of same formulation can be mixed at different proportion to produce a desired quantity of a desired strength. The strength of the mixture must lie between the strength of the stronger component and the strength of the weaker component. In the picture above 300 gram of 5% diclofenac gel (left) is being mixed with 150 gram of 8% diclofenac gel (right). The resulting mixture will be a 450 gram of 6% diclofenac gel.

Professionals working with medications use alligation calculations to manage inventory. That is, instead of making a fresh batch of a given preparation, the professional mixes the available strengths (higher and lower strength than prescribed) to arrive at the desired strength. This is only possible if the strength of the prescribed compound lies between the strengths of the available formulations.

Note: Alligation calculation is only possible with the same compound or same formulation but different strength.

In alligation calculations, two strengths are usually provided. The desired strength will usually be between the two strengths available.

The Calculation Proper

The alligation calculation is achieved using several steps. We will reveal the steps using the following example.

Example 8.1

In a pharmacy, you have enough 5% diclofenac ointment. You also have enough 12% diclofenac ointment. You receive an order to prepare 200 grams of 10% diclofenac ointment. You do not want to start making a fresh 10% diclofenac ointment but want to prepare the 10% ointment by mixing 5% and 12%. What quantities of the 5% and 12% are required to be mixed to make 200 grams of the 10%?

Solution

Available strengths = 12% and 5%

Desired strength = 10% (200 grams)

Step 1, Draw your graph for alligation calculation.

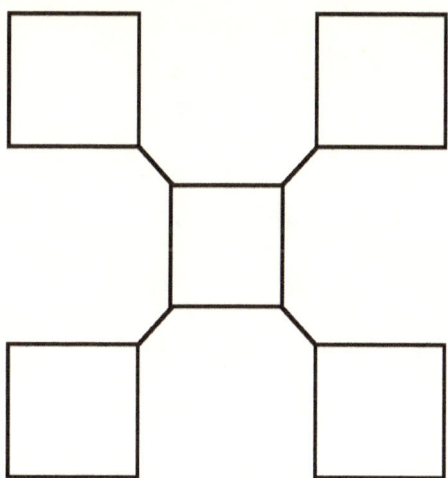

Step 2. Place the desired strength in the central box as shown in the graph.

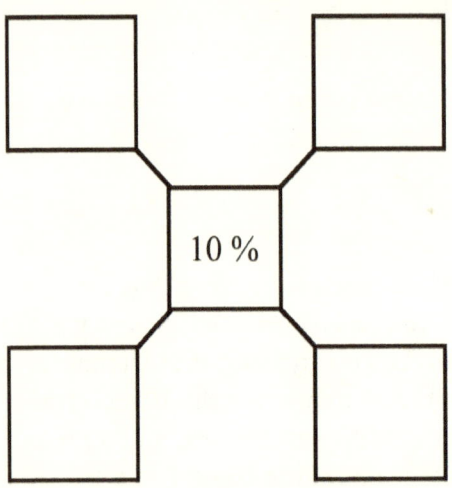

Step 3. Place the highest available percentage in the upper left corner.

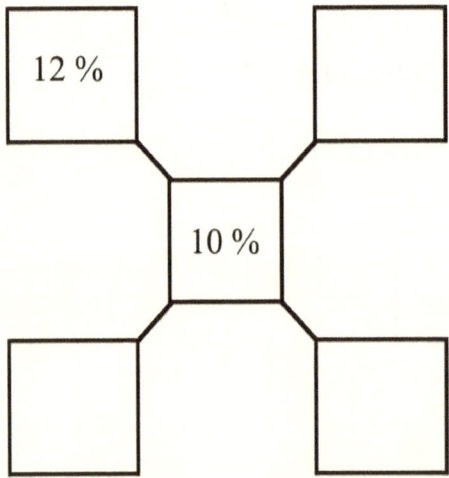

Step 4. Place the lowest available percentage in the lower-left corner.

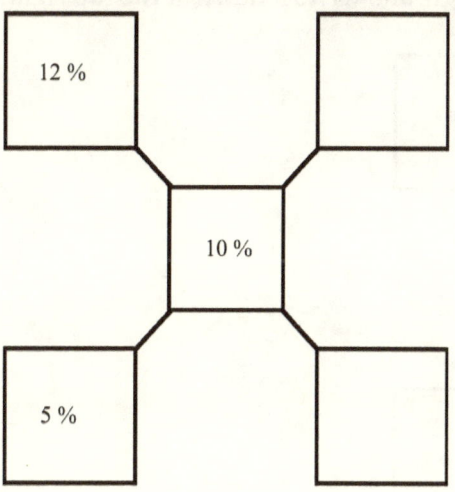

Step 5. Subtract and get the difference between the highest available strength and the desired strength, and write that down in the lower right.

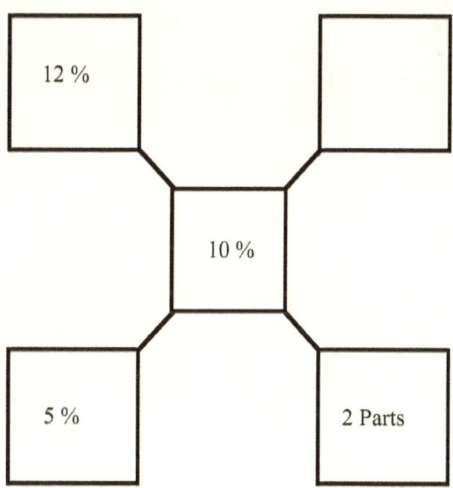

Step 6. Subtract and get the difference between the lowest available strength and the desired strength, and write it down at the top right.

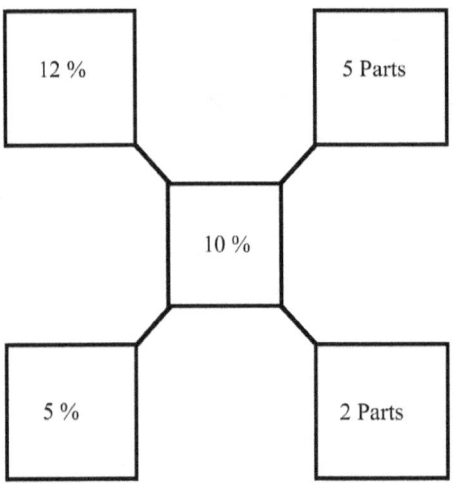

Total parts = 7

Step 7. Draw a horizontal arrow indicating the relative parts of the higher strength and the lower strength.

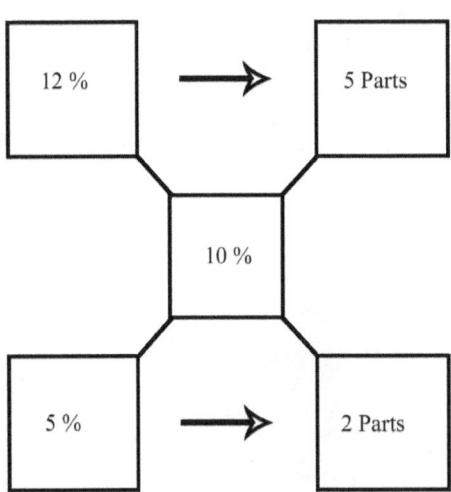

The numbers to the right (5 and 2) represent the parts of 12% and 5% respectively that are needed to make the diclofenac 10%.

That is to say: To make 10% from 12% and 5%, we need 5 parts of 12% and 2 parts of 5%.

Proportionally, it can be said that

7 grams of mixture (10%) will require 5 grams of 12%

and

7 grams of mixture (10%) will require 2 grams of 5%

That is,

$$7 \text{ g } (10\%) \rightarrow 5 \text{ g } (12\%)$$
$$7 \text{ g } (10\%) \rightarrow 2 \text{ g } (5\%)$$

Then, depending on the quantity of the new percentage desired, we can use either of the above lines of proportion as a starting point for the calculations. In the example above, the desire was to make 200 grams of the 10% strength; therefore, we can calculate the quantities of both 12% and 5% as shown below:

Calculating for the quantity of 12%

$$7 \text{ g } (10\%) \rightarrow 5 \text{ g } (12\%)$$
$$200 \text{ g } (10\%) \rightarrow u$$

$$u = \frac{5 \text{ g } (12\%)}{7 \text{ g } (10\%)} \times \frac{200 \text{ g } (10\%)}{1}$$

$$= 142.86 \text{ g } (12\%)$$

Calculating for the quantity of 5%

$$7 \text{ g } (10\%) \rightarrow 2 \text{ g } (5\%)$$
$$200 \text{ g } (10\%) \rightarrow u$$

$$u = \frac{2 \text{ g } (5\%)}{7 \text{ g } (10\%)} \times \frac{200 \text{ g } (10\%)}{1}$$

$$= 57.14 \text{ g } (5\%)$$

In other words,

200 g (10%) is achieved by mixing 142.86 g (12%) and 57.14 g (5%).

Example 8.2

How can you prepare a 2-liter solution of 30% dextrose from 50% dextrose and 20% dextrose?

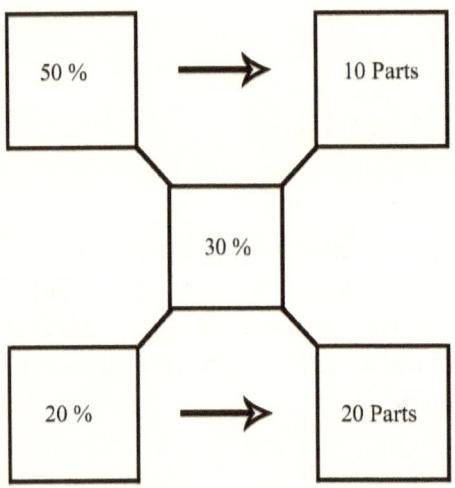

Total of parts is 20 parts + 10 parts = 30 parts

30 parts desired (30%) → 10 parts (50%) + 20 parts (20%)

Which means

30 L desired (30%) → 10 L (50%) + 20 L (20%)

Calculating for quantity of 50%

$$30 \text{ L } (30\%) \rightarrow 10 \text{ L } (50\%)$$
$$2 \text{ L } (30\%) \rightarrow u$$
$$u = \frac{10 \text{ L } (50\%)}{30 \text{ L } (30\%)} \times \frac{2 \text{ L } (30\%)}{1}$$
$$= 0.667 \text{ L } (50\%)$$

Calculating for quantity of 20%

$$30 \text{ L (30\%)} \rightarrow 20 \text{ L (20\%)}$$
$$2 \text{ L (30\%)} \rightarrow u$$

$$u = \frac{20 \text{ L (20\%)}}{30 \text{ L (30\%)}} \times \frac{2 \text{ L (30\%)}}{1}$$

$$= 1.333 \text{ L}$$

Therefore,

$$0.667 \text{ L (50\%)} + 1.333 \text{ L (20\%)}$$
$$= 2 \text{ L (30\%)}$$

Note: Always check your answer by adding the two calculated quantities of the available strength. They should equal the total quantity desired.

Example 8.3

You have 10% KCl stock solution and 60% KCl stock solution. You receive the following prescription

KCl 20% solution

M: 500 mL

How many milliliters of each solution do you need?

Solution

Available strength = 10% and 60%

Required strength = 20% (500 mL)

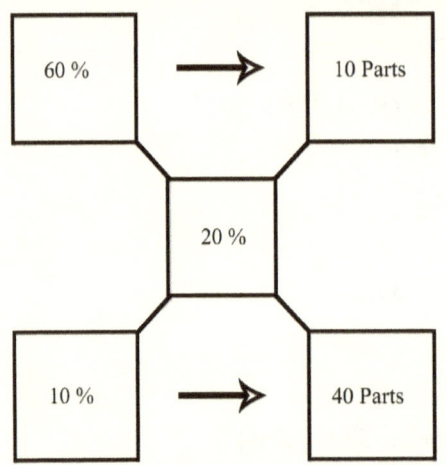

Total parts is 10 parts + 40 parts = 50 parts

50 parts desired (20%) → 10 parts (60%) + 40 parts (10%)

That is to say,

50 mL desired (20%) → 10 mL (60%) + 40 mL (10%)

Calculating for quantity of 60%

50 mL (20%) → 10 mL (60%)

500 mL (20%) → u

$$u = \frac{10 \text{ mL } (60\%)}{50 \text{ mL } (20\%)} \times \frac{500 \text{ mL } (20\%)}{1}$$

= 100 mL (60%)

Calculating for quantity of 10%

50 mL (20%) → 40 mL (10%)

500 mL (20%) → u

$$u = \frac{40 \text{ mL } (10\%)}{50 \text{ mL } (20\%)} \times \frac{500 \text{ mL } (20\%)}{1}$$

= 400 mL (10%)

100 mL (60%) + 400 mL (10%) = 500 mL (20%)

Example 8.4

You are required to prepare a 50% solution of alcohol from 70% alcohol and 20% alcohol. How many milliliters of each solution do you need to make 600 mL of the desired 50%?

Solution

Available strength = 70% and 20%

Required strength = 50% (600 mL)

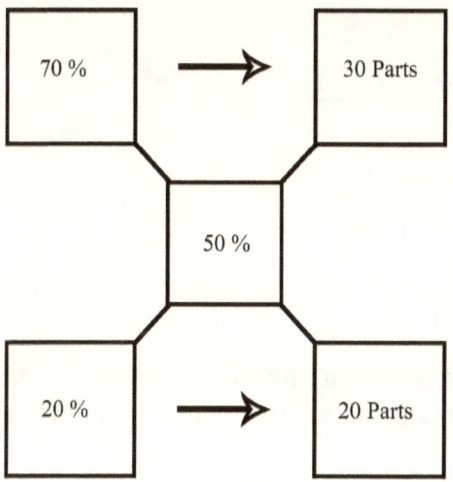

Total number of parts is 30 parts + 20 parts = 50 parts

So we can say

50 parts desired (50%) → 30 parts (70%) + 20 parts (20%)

That is to say,

50 mL desired (50%) → 30 mL (70%) + 20 mL (20%).

Calculating for quantity of 70%

$$50 \text{ mL } (50\%) \rightarrow 30 \text{ mL } (70\%)$$

$$600 \text{ mL } (50\%) \rightarrow u$$

$$u = \frac{30 \text{ mL } (70\%)}{50 \text{ mL } (50\%)} \times \frac{600 \text{ mL } (50\%)}{1}$$

$$= 360 \text{ mL of } 70\%$$

Calculating for quantity of 20%

$$50 \text{ mL } (50\%) \rightarrow 20 \text{ mL } (20\%)$$

$$600 \text{ mL } (50\%) \rightarrow u$$

$$u = \frac{20 \text{ mL } (20\%)}{50 \text{ mL } (50\%)} \times \frac{600 \text{ mL } (50\%)}{1}$$

$$= 240 \text{ mL } 20\%$$

$$360 \text{ mL } (70\%) + 240 \text{ mL } (20\%) = 600 \text{ mL } (50\%)$$

Example 8.5

You have 7.5% stock solution of potassium permanganate and 10% stock solution of potassium permanganate. You receive the following prescription:

Rx

Potassium permanganate 9%

Make 2 pints.

How many milliliters of each of the available solution do you need?

Solution

Available concentration = 7.5% and 10%

Required concentration = 9% (2 pints)

Because the answer to the question is required in milliliters, we first need to convert the 2 pints to its mL equivalent.

1 pint = 480 mL

2 pints = 480 mL × 2 = 960 mL (See chapter 2, "Interconversion of Units")

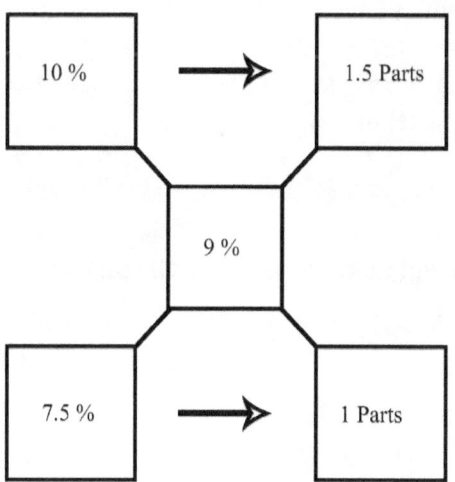

Total number of parts is 1.5 + 1 = 2.5 parts.

Therefore,

2.5 parts of the desired (9%) → 1.5 parts (10%) + 1 part (7.5%)

That is to say,

2.5 mL of the desired (9%) → 1.5 mL (10%) + 1 mL (7.5%)

Calculating for quantity of 10%

2.5 mL (9%) → 1.5 mL (10%)

960 mL (9%) → u

$$u = \frac{1.5\ mL\ (10\%)}{2.5\ mL\ (9\%)} \times \frac{960\ mL\ (9\%)}{1}$$

= 576 mL (10%)

Calculating for quantity of 7.5%

$$2.5 \text{ mL } (9\%) \rightarrow 1 \text{ mL } (7.5\%)$$
$$960 \text{ mL } (9\%) \rightarrow u$$

$$u = \frac{1 \, m \, L \, (7.5\%)}{2.5 \, ml \, (9\%)} \times \frac{960 \, mL \, (9\%)}{1}$$

$$= 384 \text{ mL } (7.5\%)$$

Therefore, when 576 mL (10%) + 384 mL (7.5%) are mixed, the resulting mixture is 960 mL (2 pints) of 9%.

Example 8.6

You have 10% dextrose solution and distilled water in the pharmacy. You received the following order:

Dextrose solution 5%

M: 900 mL

How many milliliters of the 10% and distilled water do you need to mix in order to make 900 ml of the 5%?

Solution

Available strength = 10% and 0%

Required strength = 5% (900 mL)

Note: In alligation calculations, it makes sense to consider a neutral base such as water or other diluents as zero percent because they technically contain no active ingredient in every 100 parts. It also makes sense to consider a pure drug powder or pure liquid drug as 100% because they technically contain no excipient (i.e., 100 parts of drug in every 100 parts of pure drug, which is 100%).

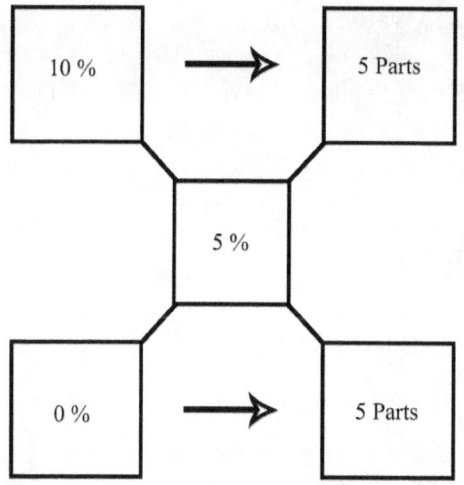

Total of parts is 5 + 5 = 10 parts.

Therefore,

      10 parts of the desired (5%) → 5 parts (10%) + 5 parts (0%).

That is to say,

      10 mL of the desired (5%) → 5 mL (10%) + 5 mL (0%).

Calculating for quantity of 10%

$$10 \text{ mL } (5\%) \rightarrow 5 \text{ mL } (10\%)$$

$$900 \text{ mL } (5\%) \rightarrow u$$

$$u = \frac{5 \text{ } mL \text{ } (10\%)}{10 \text{ } mL (5\%)} \times \frac{900 \text{ } mL \text{ } (5\%)}{1}$$

$$= 450 \text{ mL } (10\%)$$

Calculating for quantity of distilled water (0%)

$$10 \text{ mL (5\%)} \rightarrow 5 \text{ mL (distilled water)}$$

$$900 \text{ mL (5\%)} \rightarrow u$$

$$u = \frac{5 \text{ } mL \text{ } (distilled \text{ } water)}{10 \text{ } mL \text{ } (5\%)} \times \frac{900 \text{ } mL \text{ } (5\%)}{1}$$

$$= 450 \text{ mL distilled water}$$

Therefore by mixing

450 mL of 10% + 450 mL distilled water,

The result is 900 mL of 5% dextrose.

Example 8.7

You have 50% boric acid and sterile water. You receive the following prescription:

Boric acid 5%

Make 3 liters

How many milliliters of 50% boric acid and sterile water do you need?

Solution

Available strength of boric acid = 50% and 0% (sterile water contains 0% of boric acid)

Required strength = 5% (3 liters)

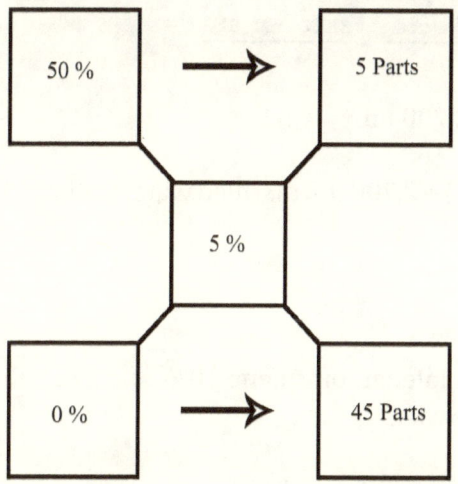

Total of parts is 5 + 45 = 50 parts

Therefore,

50 parts of the desired (5%) → 5 parts (50%) + 45 parts (0%)

That is to say,

50 mL of the desired (5%) → 5 mL (50%) + 45 mL (0%)

Calculating for quantity of 50%

$$50 \text{ mL (5\%)} \rightarrow 5 \text{ mL (50\%)}$$
$$3{,}000 \text{ mL (5\%)} \rightarrow u$$

$$u = \frac{5 \text{ mL (50\%)}}{50 \text{ mL (5\%)}} \times \frac{3{,}000 \text{ mL (5\%)}}{1}$$

$$= 300 \text{ mL (50\%)}$$

Calculating for quantity of sterile water

$$50 \text{ mL (5\%)} \rightarrow 45 \text{ mL sterile water (0\%)}$$
$$3{,}000 \text{ mL (5\%)} \rightarrow u$$

$$u = \frac{45 \; mL \; sterile \; water}{50 \; mL \; (5\%)} \times \frac{3{,}000 \; mL \; (5\%)}{1}$$

$$= 2{,}700 \; mL$$

Therefore, mixing 300 mL (50%) + 2,700 mL distilled water will yield 3,000 mL of 5%.

Example 8.8

You have an already made diclofenac ointment 10% and enough quantities of pure diclofenac powder.

You receive the following prescription from the physician:

> Diclofenac 12.5% ointment
>
> AAA BID to thigh muscles
>
> M: 300 grams

What quantities of the 10% and the pure diclofenac powder will you mix to arrive at the desired quantity of 12.5%?

Solution

Note: Pure powder drug substance is considered to be 100% (because there is 100 grams of drug in 100 grams of powder heap).

Available strength = 10% and 100%

Required strength = 12.5% (300 g)

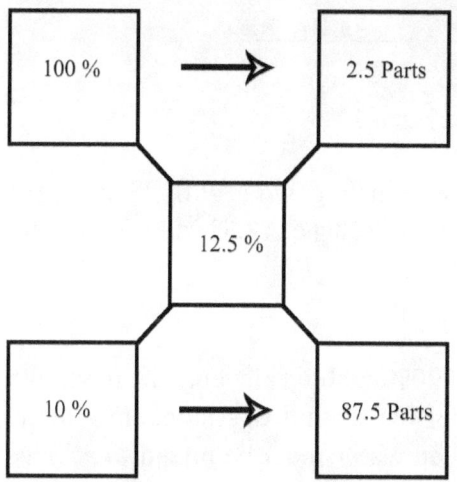

Total of parts is 2.5 + 87.5 = 90 parts

Therefore,

> 90 parts of the desired (12.5%) → 2.5
> parts (100%) + 87.5 parts (10%)

That is to say,

> 90 g of the desired (12.5%) → 2.5 g (100%) + 87.5 g (10%)

Calculating for quantity of pure powder

> 90 g (12.5%) → 2.5 g diclo powder (100%)
>
> 300 g (12.5%) → u

$$u = \frac{2.5 \ g \ diclo \ powder}{90 \ g \ (12.5\%)} \times \frac{300 \ g \ (12.5\%)}{1}$$

> = 8.333 g diclo powder

Calculating for quantity of 10%

> 90 g (12.5%) → 87.5 g (10%)
>
> 300 g (12.5%) → u

$$u = \frac{87.5\,g(10\%)}{90\,g\,(12.5\%)} \times \frac{300\,g\,(12.5\%)}{1}$$

$$= 291.667 \text{ g of } 10\%$$

Therefore, by blending 8.333 g pure diclo powder with 291.667 g of 10% diclo ointment, the result will be 300 g of 12.5% diclo ointment.

Example 8.9

A hospital has a stock solution of 90% rubbing alcohol. The physician ordered 180 mL of 70% alcohol for wound dressing. How many milliliters of the 90% and distilled water must be mixed to achieve the 70% alcohol?

Solution

Available strength = 90% alcohol and 0% alcohol (distilled water)

Required strength = 70% alcohol (180 mL)

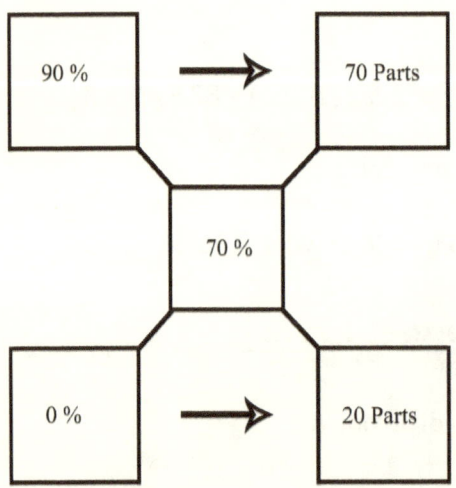

Total of parts is 70 + 20 = 90 parts

Therefore,

90 parts of the desired (70%) → 70 parts (90%) + 20 part (0%)

That is to say,

90 mL of the desired (70%) → 70 mL (90%) + 20 mL (0%)

Calculation for quantity of 90%

90 mL (70%) → 70 mL (90%)

180 mL (70%) → u

$$u = \frac{70 \ mL \ (90\%)}{90 \ mL \ (70\%)} \times \frac{180 \ mL \ (70\%)}{1}$$

= 140 mL (90%)

Calculating for quantity of distilled water

90 mL (70%) → 20 mL distilled water (0%)

180 mL (70%) → u

$$u = \frac{20 \ mL \ distilled \ water}{90 \ mL \ (70\%)} \times \frac{180 \ mL \ (70\%)}{1}$$

= 40 mL distilled water

Therefore, mixing 140 mL (90%) + 40 mL distilled water will yield 180 mL of the desired 70% alcohol.

Example 8.10

You have already made 10% lidocaine in Diffusimax. You also have enough plain Diffusimax in the pharmacy. You receive the following order:

Lidocaine 6% in Diffusimax

Apply to affected area UD

Make 500 g

How many grams of 10% and plain Diffusimax are needed to be mixed to make the 500 g of the 6%?

Solution

Available strength = 10% and 0% (plain Diffusimax contains no lidocaine)

Required strength = 6% (500 grams)

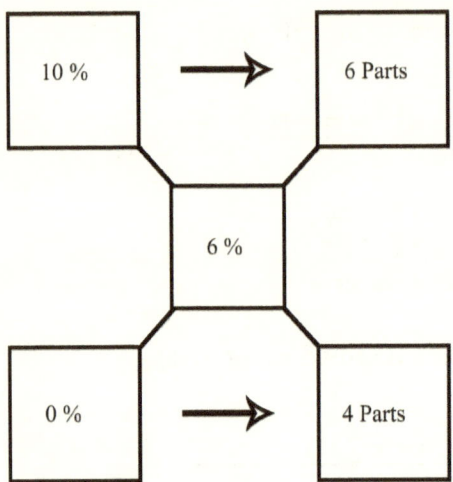

Total of parts is 6 + 4 = 10 parts.

Therefore,

10 parts of the desired (6%) → 6 parts (10%) + 4 parts (0%)

That is to say,

10 g of the desired (6%) → 6 g (10%) + 4 g (0%)

Calculating for quantity of 10%

10 g (6%) → 6 g lidocaine (10%)

500 g (6%) → u

$$u = \frac{6\ g\ lidocaine(10\%)}{10\ g\ (6\%)} \times \frac{500\ g\ (6\%)}{1}$$

= 300 g 10% lidocaine

Calculating for quantity of Diffusimax (0%)

$$10 \text{ g } (6\%) \rightarrow 4 \text{ g Diffusimax } (0\%)$$

$$500 \text{ g } (6\%) \rightarrow u$$

$$u = \frac{4 \text{ g } Diffusimax\,(0\%)}{10g\ (6\%)} \times \frac{500 \text{ g } (6\%)}{1}$$

$$= 200 \text{ g Diffusimax } (0\%)$$

Therefore, blending 300 g of 10% lidocaine + 200 g of plain Diffusimax = 500 g of 6% lidocaine in Diffusimax.

Example 8.11

You want to make 800 mL of 20% potassium permanganate from your stock of 5% and 70% potassium permanganate. You discovered that only 150 mL of 70% potassium permanganate is available. What is the maximum volume of the 20% you can make with the available stock 150 mL of 70%?

Solution

Available strength = 70% and 5%

Required strength = 20% (800 mL)

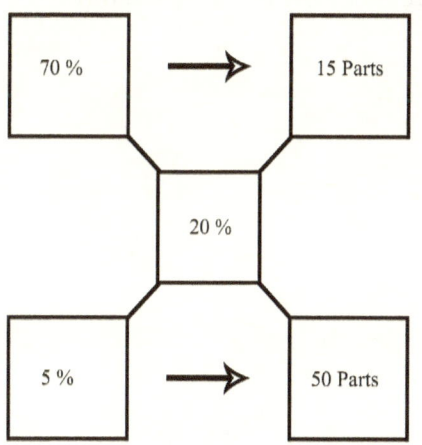

70 %   15 Parts

20 %

5 %   50 Parts

Total part is 15 + 50 = 65 parts

Therefore,

65 parts of the desired (20%) → 50 parts (5%) + 15 parts (70%)

That is to say,

65 mL of the desired (20%) → 50 mL (5%) + 15 mL (70%)

It follows that 65 mL of 20% will be produced using 15 mL of 70%

That is,

65 mL (20%) → 15 mL (70%)

Now we are calculating for the volume of 20% given the limited availability of the 70%. Our line of proportionality will be reversed to have the volume of 20% on the right. Thus

15 mL (70%) → 65 mL (20%)

150 mL (70%) → u

$$u = \frac{65 \ mL \ (20\%)}{15 \ mL \ (70\%)} \times \frac{150 \ mL \ (70\%)}{1}$$

= 650 mL

We simply need 150 mL (70%) + 500 mL of 5% to make 650 mL of the desired 20%.

Chapter 8 Practice Questions

1. You have 5% diclofenac gel and 12% diclofenac gel. You receive an order to make 200 grams of 8%.

   - How many grams of 5% are needed?
   - How many grams of 12% are needed?

2. You want to prepare 8% potassium permanganate solution from 5% and 15%. You discovered you have enough of 15% solution but only 80 mL of the 5% solution. What is the maximum volume of the potassium permanganate you can make?

3. You have in stock minoxidil 4% in CeraVe cream. You also have in stock enough of minoxidil powder. You receive a prescription of 300 gram of minoxidil 10% in CeraVe.

   - How many grams of minoxidil 4% will be needed?

   - How many grams of pure minoxidil powder will be needed?

4. You have hydrocortisone ointment (2% and 1%) stock. You received the following prescription:

   Hydrocortisone ointment 1.8%
   Make 300 g

   - How many grams of 1% are needed?
   - How many grams of 2% will be needed?

5. You have in the pharmacy 5% Lysol solution and 15% Lysol solution. You are required to make 400 mL of 7% Lysol solution.

   - How many milliliters of 5% Lysol will be needed?
   - How many milliliters of 15% Lysol solution will be needed?

6. You are required to prepare 4.4 pounds of 5.6% menthol ointment. The available menthol ointments are 2.7% and 12%.

   - How many grams of 2.7% menthol ointment will be needed?
   - How many grams of 12% menthol ointment will be needed?

7. You are required to prepare two cups of isotonic solution (0.9% sodium chloride) using 2% sodium chloride and 0.5% sodium chloride solution.

   - How many milliliters of the 0.5% solution will be needed?
   - How many milliliters of the 2% solution will be needed?

8. You received the following order:

   Alcohol solution 50%
   Make 2 gallons

   You have available 30% alcohol solution and 70% alcohol solution.

   - How many milliliters of 30% alcohol will be needed?
   - How many milliliters of 70% alcohol will be needed?

9. You receive the following physician's order:

   Burow's solution 7.5%
   Make 800 mL

You have in stock a 25% Burow's solution and sterile water.

- How many milliliters of sterile water will be needed?
- How many milliliters of 25% Burow's solution will be needed?

10. You receive the following prescription:

Diclofenac 8% in Diffusimax
Make 100 grams

In your pharmacy, you have already made 10% diclofenac in Diffusimax. You also have plain Diffusimax.

- How many grams of Diffusimax will be needed?
- How many grams of 10% diclofenac will be needed?

11. You receive the following prescription:
Diclofenac 12% in PLO gel
Apply UD
    Make 300 g

You have 10% diclofenac already made and enough quantity of pure diclofenac powder.

- How many grams of 10% will be needed?
- How many grams of pure diclofenac powder will be needed?

12. You have enough 20% menthol ointment available but only 50 grams of 5% menthol ointment. What is the maximum amount of 12% menthol ointment you can make?

13. Prepare 500 mL of 10% Lysol solution using 50% Lysol solution and distilled water.

    - How many milliliters of distilled water will be needed?
    - How many milliliters of 10% Lysol solution will be needed?

14. A physician orders the following:

    Boric acid ointment 16%
    AAA TID PRN
        M: 0.88 pounds

    Available are two boric acid ointments in 12% and 24% strengths in the pharmacy.

    - How many grams of 12% will be needed?
    - How many grams of 24% will be needed?

15. How do you prepare 1,960 grams of 5% gabapentin ointment from 2% gabapentin ointment and pure gabapentin powder?

    - How many grams of 2% gabapentin ointment will be needed?
    - How many grams of pure gabapentin powder will be needed?

16. A physician orders 40 grams of 12% boric acid ointment. You have enough of 25% and only 10 g of 10%. What is the maximum quantity of the 10% you can make?

17. A physician wants 100 grams of an 8% ointment. The available stock ointments are 5% and 12%.

    - How many grams of 5% will be needed?
    - How many grams of 12% will be needed?

18. Prepare 300 mL of 8% dextrose solution for IV administration using distilled water and 20% dextrose.

- How many milliliters of distilled water will be needed?
- How many milliliters of 20% will be needed?

19. On hand is 50 mL of 6% dextrose solution and enough of 15% dextrose solution. You want to prepare a 10% solution of dextrose. What is the maximum volume of the 10% you can make?

20. Available are two menthol ointment strengths of 5% menthol and 20% menthol. You are required to make a compound of menthol based on the following prescription:

Menthol ointment 18%
Apply UD
    M: 0.4 kg

- How many grams of 5% menthol ointment will be needed?
- How many grams of 20% menthol ointment will be needed?

21. Consider the following prescription:

Gabapentin 10% in Aquaphor
Apply to feet QID UD
    M: 200 grams

You have 6% gabapentin in Aquaphor already made and enough gabapentin powder. You want to make the 10% gabapentin using the stock 6% and the gabapentin powder.

- How many grams of 6% gabapentin will be needed?
- How many grams of gabapentin powder will be needed?

22. You have available 10% lidocaine in PLO gel and 6% lidocaine in PLO gel. You receive an order to make 1.76 pounds of 7% lidocaine in PLO gel.

    - How many grams of 6% lidocaine will be needed?
    - How many grams of 10% lidocaine will be needed?

23. You have available in the pharmacy 1.5% potassium chloride solution and 5% potassium chloride solution. You receive the following order:

    Potassium chloride solution 3%
        Prepare 3 pints

    - How many milliliters of 1.5% solution will be needed?
    - How many milliliters of 5% solution will be needed?

24. You have 3% hydrocortisone cream in Dermabase. Physician prescribes 80 grams of a 1% hydrocortisone in Dermabase to treat eczema for an infant. You want to make the 1% hydrocortisone by diluting the 3% with neutral base (Dermabase).

    - How many grams of the Dermabase will be needed?
    - How many grams of 3% cream will be needed?

25. You set out to prepare 300 grams of cyclobenzaprine 10% in Eucerin base. You have in stock 6% cyclobenzaprine in Eucerin base and enough cyclobenzaprine powder.

    - How many grams of 6% cyclobenzaprine preparation will be needed?
    - How many grams of pure cyclobenzaprine powder will be needed?

26. You have 5% KCl solution and 15% KCl solution, and you are required to make 500 mL of 12% KCl solution.

    -   How many milliliters of 5% solution are needed?
    -   How many milliliters of 15% solution are needed?

27. A physician orders 22 pounds of a 7.5% cream. The available strengths of the cream are 2.5% and 20%.

    -   How many grams of 2.5% cream will be needed?
    -   How many grams of 20% cream will be needed?

28. You receive the following order:

    Dextrose solution 20%
        Make 2 L

    Available in the pharmacy, you have distilled water and a 50% dextrose solution.

    -   How many milliliters of the distilled water are needed?
    -   How many milliliters of the 50% solution are needed?

29. Available in the pharmacy, you have dextrose 5% solution and dextrose 50% solution. You receive the following physician's order:

    For dextrose solution 7%
        Make 5 cups

    -   How many milliliters of 5% solution are needed?
    -   How many milliliters of 50% solution are needed?

30. You only have in the pharmacy 20% potassium permanganate and sterile water. You received an order to prepare 4 cups of 12% potassium permanganate solution.

- How many milliliters of the sterile water will be needed?
- How many milliliters of 20% solution will be needed?

31. Available in the pharmacy are 8% diclofenac ointment and 10% diclofenac ointment. You received the following prescription:

Diclofenac 9%
Apply UD
　　M: 0.45 kg

- How many grams of 8% will be needed?
- How many grams of 10% will be needed?

32. You have 50% salicylic acid in Vaseline and enough quantity of plain Vaseline in the pharmacy. You receive the following physician's order:

Salicylic acid 20%
　　Make 200 grams

- How many grams of Vaseline will be needed?
- How many grams of 50% salicylic acid will be needed?

33. You receive a prescription to make 250 grams of 10% strength of a certain ointment. You have in stock the highest strength of the ointment, precisely 15%. You also have the neutral base in stock.

- How many grams of the 15% stock ointment will be needed?
- How many grams of the neutral base will be needed?

34. You intend to prepare 500 mL of 8% dextrose solution from 10% and 5% dextrose solution. You just discovered you had enough of 10% but only 60 mL of 5%. What is the maximum volume of the 8% you can prepare?

35. You have 90% alcohol available and 50% alcohol also available. You are required to make 200 mL of 80% alcohol.

   - How many milliliters of 50% alcohol solution will be needed?
   - How many milliliters of 90% alcohol solution will be needed?

36. You receive the following order:

   Potassium permanganate 3%
       Make 25 oz

   You have available 8% potassium permanganate and 2% potassium permanganate.

   - How many milliliters of 2% will be needed?
   - How many milliliters of 8% will be needed?

37. You have only 50% boric acid solution and distilled water in the pharmacy. You receive the following emergency order:

   Boric acid solution 20%
       Make 1 L

   - How many milliliters of distilled water will be needed?
   - How many milliliters of 50% will be needed?

38. A 5% dextrose solution is available in the hospital, as well as a 50% dextrose solution. You receive the following order:

Dextrose 10%
For intravenous administration
     500 mL

-   How many milliliters of 5% will be needed?
-   How many milliliters of 50% will be needed?

39. In the pharmacy, you have gabapentin 30% cream in Glaxal base. You also have enough plain Glaxal base in stock. You receive the following physician's order:

Gabapentin 6% in Glaxal base
     Make 300 grams

-   How many grams of Glaxal base will be needed?
-   How many grams of gabapentin 30% will be needed?

40. You have on hand 6% potassium permanganate solution and 15% potassium permanganate. You are required to prepare 1.5 pints of 10% potassium permanganate.

-   How many milliliters of 6% will be needed?
-   How many milliliters of 15% will be needed?

41. You have 7% clindamycin cream and 13% clindamycin cream. You receive the following order:

Clindamycin cream 11%
     Make 120 grams

-   How many grams of 7% will be needed?
-   How many grams of 13% will be needed

42. Compound a 3.8% solution from 12% stock solution and distilled water for a total volume of 2.5 pints. How many milliliters of distilled water and the 12% do you need?

43. Prepare 7 oz of 6% potassium permanganate solution from 45% stock solution and sterile water. How many milliliters of the 45% solution and the sterile water are needed?

44. Compound 450 grams of clindamycin cream 12% from 5% cream and pure clindamycin powder. How many grams of each are needed for the compound?

45. You have a stock solution of 30% and 20%. How much of each do you need to make 8 ounces of 22% solution?

46. How many grams of petrolatum should be mixed with what amount in grams of 15% cyclobenzaprine ointment (in petrolatum) in order to produce 480 g of 10% cyclobenzaprine ointment?

47. You have 8% menthol cream and 12% menthol cream. You receive the following order:

10% menthol cream
    Make 150 grams

- How many grams of 8% will be needed?
- How many grams of 12% will be needed

48. In the pharmacy, you have 3% hydrocortisone cream in Glaxal base. You also have enough plain Glaxal base in stock. You receive the following physician's order:

2.5% hydrocortisone in Glaxal base
    Make 400 grams

- How many grams of Glaxal base will be needed?
- How many grams of 3% hydrocortisone will be needed?

49. You have only 20% tannic acid solution and distilled water in the pharmacy. You receive the following emergency order:

Tannic acid solution 7.5%
    Make 8 cups

- How many liters of distilled water will be needed?
- How many liters of 20% will be needed?

50. You received an order for 500 grams of 12.5% diclofenac gel. You have enough ready-made 10% diclofenac and enough diclofenac powder in store. How much of the two ingredients will you need to make the desired percentage and quantity?

★ Star Question ★

Two different strengths of ranitidine suspension 2 % and 2.5% are mixed together in the ratio of 4:5 to make a total volume of 270 ml of a homogeneous ranitidine suspension mixture.

How many mLs of this mixture should be given to a child as a single dose with the following prescription?

Ranitidine 4mg/kg/dose

Patient weighs 52.8 pounds

Answers to Chapter 8
Practice Questions

1. 85.71 g of 12%
   114.29 g of 5%
2. 114.29 mL
3. 281.25 g of 4%
   18.75 g of minoxidil powder
4. 60 g of 1%
   240 g of 2%
5. 320 mL of 5%
   80 mL of 15%
6. 1,376.34 g of 2.7%
   623.66 g of 12%
7. 352 mL of 0.5%
   128 mL of 2%
8. 3,840 mL of 30%
   3,840 mL of 70%
9. 560 mL of sterile water
   240 mL of 25%
10. 20 g of plain Diffusimax
    80 g of 10%
11. 293.33 g of 10%
    6.67 g of pure diclofenac powder
12. 93.75 g
13. 400 mL distilled water
    100 mL of 50%
14. 266.67 g of 12%
    133.33 g of 24%
15. 1,900 g of 2%
    60 g of pure gabapentin powder
16. 11.54 g
17. 57.143 g of 5%
    42.857 g of 12%
18. 180 mL of distilled water

120 mL of 20%
19. 90 mL
20. 53.33 g of 5%
346.67 g of 20%
21. 191.49 g of 6%
8.51 g of pure gabapentin powder
22. 600 g of 6%
200 g of 10%
23. 822.86 g of 1.5%
617.14 g of 5%
24. 53.33 g of Dermabase
26.67 g of 3%
25. 287.23 g of 6%
12.77 g of cyclobenzaprine powder
26. 150 mL of 5%
350 mL of 15%
27. 7,142.86 g of 2.5%
2,875.14 g 20%
28. 1,200 mL of distilled water
800 mL of 50%
29. 1,146.67 mL of 5%
53.33 mL of 50%
30. 384 mL sterile water
576 mL of 20%
31. 225 g of 8%
225 g of 10%
32. 120 g of Vaseline
80 g of 50%
33. 83.33 g neutral base
166.67 g of 15%
34. 150 mL
35. 50 mL of 50%
150 mL of 90%
36. 625 mL of 2%
125 mL of 8%
37. 600 mL distilled water
400 mL of 50%

38. 444.44 mL of 5%
    55.56 mL of 50%
39. 240 g of Glaxal base
    60 g of 30%
40. 400 mL of 6%
    320 mL of 15%
41. 40 g of 7%
    80 g of 13%
42. 820 mL distilled water
    380 mL 12%
43. 182 mL of sterile water
    28 mL of 45%
44. 416.84 g of 5%
    33.16 g of pure clindamycin powder
45. 192 mL of 20%
    48 mL of 30%
46. 160 g of petrolatum
    320 g of 15%
47. 75 g of 8%
    75 g of 12%
48. 66.67 g of Glaxal base
    333.33 g of 3%
49. 1.2 L distilled water
    0.72 L of 20%
50. 486.11 g of 10%
    13.89 g of pure diclofenac powder

Solution to the star question

First calculate the respective volumes contributed by the different strength of the ranitidine suspension. Total volume of the mixture comes from the volume contributed by the 2% suspension and the volume contributed by the 2.5% suspension.

The ratio 4:5 means that the 2% suspension contributed 4 parts to the volume while the 2.5% contributed 5 parts to the entire volume, making a total of 9 parts.

4 parts (2%) + 5 parts (2.5%) = 9 parts mixture

That is,

9 parts (mixture) → 4 parts (2%) + 5 parts (2.5%)

This also means that

9 mL (mixture) → 4 mL (2%) + 5 mL (2.5%)

The proportional equation above can be used to determine the individual contribution to the volume of 270 mL

Calculating for the volume of the 2%

9 mL (mixture) → 4 mL (2%)

270 mL (mixture) → u

$$u = \frac{4 \text{ mL (2\%)}}{9 \text{ mL (mixture)}} \times \frac{270 \text{ mL (mixture)}}{1}$$

= 120 mL of 2%

Calculating for the volume of the 2.5%

9 mL (mixture) → 5 mL (2.5%)

270 mL (mixture) → u

$$u = \frac{5 \text{ mL (2.5\%)}}{9 \text{ mL (mixture)}} \quad \text{X} \quad \frac{270 \text{ mL (mixture)}}{1}$$

=150 mL of 2.5%

Therefore the 2% contributed 120 mL while the 2.5% contributed 150 ml and both contributions made up the 270 ml of the mixture.

Next, determine the amount of the active ingredient that was contributed by each strength.

For the 2% suspension (120 mL)

2% means that every 100 mL of the suspension contains 2 gram of ranitidine. How many grams will be contained in the 120 mL?

100 mL suspension → 2 g ranitidine

120 mL suspension → u

$$u = \frac{2 \text{ g ranitidine}}{100 \text{ mL suspension}} \quad \text{X} \quad \frac{120 \text{ mL suspension}}{1}$$

= 2.4 gram ranitidine

For the 2.5% suspension (150 mL)

2.5% means that every 100 mL of the suspension contains 2.5 gram of ranitidine. How many grams will be contained in the 150 mL?

100 mL suspension → 2.5 g ranitidine

150 mL suspension → u

$$u = \frac{2.5 \text{ g ranitidine}}{100 \text{ mL suspension}} \times \frac{150 \text{ mL suspension}}{1}$$

= 3.75 gram ranitidine

So the 2% contributed 2.4 grams of ranitidine to the mixture while the 2.5% contributed 3.75 grams of ranitidine to the mixture. The total amount of ranitidine in the mixture will be

2.4 g + 3.75 g = 6.15 g ranitidine

It can be said that 6.15 gram of ranitidine is contained in the 270 ml of the mixture.

Dosage calculations

Weight of the child is 52.8 pounds

This weight should be converted to kg since the child's dosage is expressed in kg.

2.2 pounds → 1 kg

52.8 pounds → u

$$u = \frac{1 \text{ kg}}{2.2 \text{ pounds}} \times \frac{52.8 \text{ pounds}}{1}$$

= 24 kg

The dosage of 4 mg/kg per dose means that the child should receive 4 mg ranitidine for every kilogram body weight per dose

 1 kg body weight → 4 mg ranitidine

24 kg body weight → u

$$u = \frac{4 \text{ mg ranitidine}}{1 \text{ kg body weight}} \times \frac{24 \text{ kg body weight}}{1}$$

= 96 mg ranitidine per dose.

But how many mLs of the mixture should that be if 6.15 gram of ranitidine is contained in 270 ml of the mixture?

6.15 gram is equivalent to 6150 mg (see chapter 2, interconversion of units)

6150 mg ranitidine → 270 ml mixture

 96 mg ranitidine → u

$$u = \frac{270 \text{ mL mixture}}{6150 \text{ mg ranitidine}} \times \frac{96 \text{ mg ranitidine}}{1}$$

= 4.215 mL approx.

CHAPTER 9

Calculations Involving Dilutions of Formulations

Introduction

Sometimes, in order to fill a prescription order from a prescriber, a medical professional may be confronted with the challenge of simply diluting an existing highly concentrated formulation to a lower concentration in accordance with the requirements of the medication order. For example, if the pharmacy has a stock solution of 20% boric acid and a prescription order calls for a certain volume of 5% boric acid, by careful calculations, a certain volume of diluent must definitely be added to a certain volume of the 20% boric acid to achieve both the desired strength (5%) and the desired volume.

When prescriptions are written for a liquid or a solid/semisolid medication that is not commercially available in the strength prescribed, the pharmacist utilizes dilution and concentration calculations to proceed. In most cases, the stock concentration (or available commercial strength) is higher than the prescribed strength. In this situation, the available strength must be diluted by the medical professional in order to lower the strength. This is called dilution.

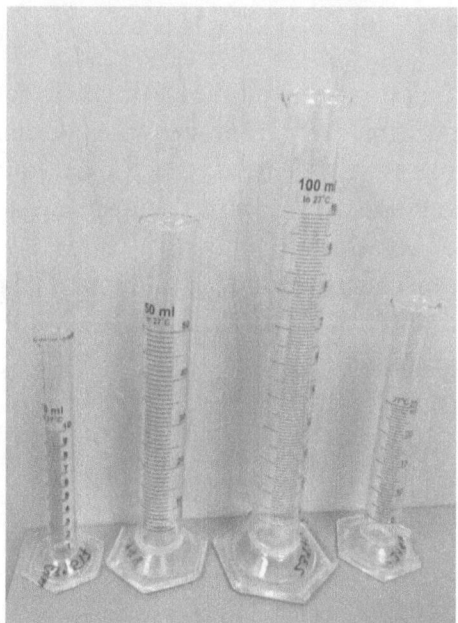

FIGURE 9.1 *The Measuring Cylinders:* These are simple equipment for volume measurement (usually calibrated in mL) and they come in different shapes and capacities. With the measuring cylinders, specific volumes of liquid preparations, vehicles and diluents are measured.

Dilution is therefore the process of adding a certain amount of diluent or solvent to a certain amount of stock solution or formulation in order to arrive at a certain volume of a lower concentration of the same formulation. The diluent (or solvent) is an inert substance with zero concentration and can be considered a neutral base or vehicle. The diluent adds either volume or mass to the preparation and thereby lowers the strength of the preparation.

The desire to lower the strength of an existing preparation (dilution) is more common than the desire to increase the strength (concentration) of an existing preparation. To increase the concentration of a preparation will involve the careful addition of the active ingredient to the available preparation or evaporation of volatile diluent from a preparation. In this book, we will place our emphasis on dilution rather than concentration.

The Dilution Equation

Whenever a formulation with an initial concentration, C_1, and initial quantity of formulation, Q_1, is diluted by the addition of an inactive diluent, leading to a new (lower) concentration, C_2, and a new (bigger) quantity of formulation, Q_2, it is a fact that the product of the initial concentration (C_1) and the initial quantity (Q_1) is always equal to the product of the final concentration (C_2) and the final quantity (Q_2) so long as the two concentrations (C_1 and C_2) are of the same type of concentration expression.

That is to say,

$$C_1 \times Q_1 = C_2 \times Q_2$$
$$C_1 Q_1 = C_2 Q_2$$

Where:

C_1 = Initial concentration
Q_1 = Initial quantity of formulation
C_2 = Final concentration
Q_2 = Final quantity of formulation

In the dilution process, C_1 is always higher than C_2 while Q_2 is always obviously bigger than Q_1.

It is beyond the scope of this book to prove this equation.

If 60 mL of a 5% solution of a liquid formulation is diluted to 100 mL, the resulting concentration of the diluted solution would be 3%.

$$C_1 Q_1 = C_2 Q_2$$
$$5 \times 60 = 3 \times 100 = 300$$

When three components of this equation are provided in a question, the fourth component can easily be calculated by simple mathematical manipulation. Most calculations surrounding dilutions can be accomplished using this formula.

In this book, however, there is de-emphasis on the use of formulas. The target of this book is to ground the students on the fundamental principles that play a part in proportional pharmaceutical calculations.

Students are recommended to review the chapter on expressions of concentrations (chapter 4) where different ways of expressing concentrations have been described. This chapter will involve interconversion of concentration from one form to another and therefore demands proper understanding of each concentration expression.

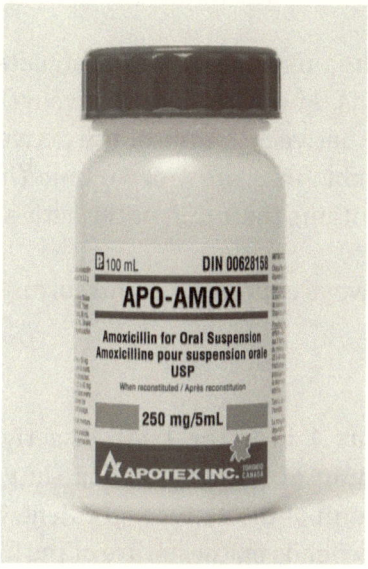

FIGURE 9.2 *Dilution by Reconstitution:* The simplest form of dilution is to add a specified amount of distilled water to a dry powdered formulation as recommended in the product insert. For example, adding a specified amount of distilled water into one bottle of Apo-amoxicillin dry powder will produce a suspension ready for administration. This form of dilution is called reconstitution. Manufacturers prepare some medication as dry powder in order to reduce the cost of transportation by weight and more importantly improve the shelf life of the product. Most reconstituted formulations are required to be discarded some days after reconstitution. (Courtesy APOTEX)

The concentration of a pharmaceutical formulation can be expressed in either of three ways.

Percentage strength (%) expresses the amount of active ingredients in grams or milliliters contained in every 100 grams or 100 mL of the formulation (depending on the nature of active ingredient and the formulation). A solution of 1% prednisolone contains 1 gram of prednisolone in every 100 mL of the solution.

Note: In percentage strength, the amount of active ingredient is expressed in grams (not milligrams) or milliliters if pure ingredient is available as liquid, and the amount of formulation is expressed in grams (for weighable preparations) and milliliters for liquid preparations.

The ratio strength is used mainly to designate the concentration of weak preparations. At a glance, ratio strength expression shows clearly the relation between 1 unit of the active ingredient (1 g or 1 mL) and the weight (in grams) or volume (in milliliters) of the preparation that contains the 1 unit of the active ingredient.

Ratio strength is always expressed in this form:

$$1:x$$

Where '1' represents 1 gram or 1 mL of active ingredient and x represents the amount of the formulation (in grams or milliliters) that contains the 1 unit of the active ingredient. The unit of measure of the formulation depends on the nature of the formulation. The unit will be gram if the formulation is such that is weighable, while the unit of the preparation will be in milliliters if the preparation is one of liquid consistency.

For example, 1:1,000 ratio strength of epinephrine solution means that every 1,000 mL of the solution will contain 1 gram of pure epinephrine.

Note: The unit of measure for the '1' in ratio strength is gram or milliliters depending on the nature of the active ingredient.

The fractional concentration expression clearly shows the amount of the active ingredient per unit amount of the formulation. For example, a 5 mg/3 mL suspension means that each 3 mL of the formulation should contain 5 mg of the active ingredient. This method of expressing concentration makes it easier to see at first instance how much of the active ingredient is contained per unit of the preparation.

By using proportion principles, various calculations involving dilution can be performed. We must realize that after dilution, the final concentration must be lower than the initial concentration, and the final quantity of formulation will be bigger than the starting quantity because some diluents had been added to dilute the stock during the process of the dilutions.

Example 9.1

How many grams of boric acid are contained in 400 mL of 10% boric acid solution?

Solution

The solution to this problem begins from proper understanding of the meaning of the percentage provided.

A 10% solution of boric acid means that every 100 mL of the solution contains 10 grams of boric acid. This will form the base of our logic for proportional calculation as we search for the amount of boric acid that will be contained in 400 mL of the boric acid solution.

$$100 \text{ mL solution} \rightarrow 10 \text{ g boric acid}$$

$$400 \text{ mL solution} \rightarrow u$$

$$u = \frac{10 \text{ g boric acid}}{100 \text{ mL solution}} \times \frac{400 \text{ mL solution}}{1}$$

$$= 40 \text{ g boric acid}$$

Example 9.2

How many grams of epinephrine are contained in 200 mL of a 1:1,000 epinephrine solution?

Solution

In this problem, we need to first understand what the ratio strength stands for. A 1:1,000 solution of epinephrine simply means that every 1,000 mL of the epinephrine solution contains 1 gram of the pure epinephrine. This concept will form our basis for the calculation of the amount of epinephrine that will be contained in 200 mL of the solution.

$$1{,}000 \text{ mL epinephrine solution} \rightarrow 1 \text{ g epinephrine}$$

$$200 \text{ mL epinephrine solution} \rightarrow u$$

$$u = \frac{1 \text{ g epinephrine}}{1{,}000 \text{ mL epinephrine solution}} \times \frac{200 \text{ mL epinephrine solution}}{1}$$

$$= 0.2 \text{ g epinephrine}$$

Therefore, 200 mL of 1:1,000 epinephrine solution will contain 0.2 grams of epinephrine.

Example 9.3

After adding the required amount of distilled water to amoxicillin powder for reconstitution, the concentration will become 250 mg/5mL. The dentist's order requires 2 grams of amoxicillin to be administered to a patient one hour prior to dental appointment. How many milliliters of the suspension should be administered to the patient?

Solution

It is clear from the strength of the amoxicillin suspension that every 5 mL of the suspension must contain 250 mg of amoxicillin (active ingredient). This will form the basis for the calculation of the volume that will deliver 2 grams of the active ingredient to the patient.

250 mg amoxicillin → 5 mL suspension

2 g amoxicillin → u

Note: We keep the mL to the right-hand side of the line of proportion because we are looking for the mL. See Chapter 1 for rules of proportion calculation.

Looking at the left-hand side of the lines of proportion, we will quickly observe that the two units of weight (250 mg and 2 g) are not the same; therefore, our calculation cannot proceed according to our guiding rules (chapter 1). Hence, one of the units must be converted to the other in order to proceed. We therefore need to convert the gram to its milligram equivalent. Thus

$$1 \text{ g} \rightarrow 1,000 \text{ mg}$$

$$2 \text{ g} \rightarrow u$$

$$u = \frac{1,000 \text{ mg}}{1 \text{ g}} \times \frac{2 \text{ g}}{1}$$

$$= 2,000 \text{ mg}$$

(see chapter 2, "Interconversion of Units")

Continuing with our earlier calculation

250 **mg** amoxicillin → 5 mL suspension

2,000 **mg** amoxicillin → u

$$u = \frac{5 \text{ mL suspension}}{250 \text{ mg amoxicillin}} \times \frac{2,000 \text{ mg amoxicillin}}{1}$$

$$= 40 \text{ mL}$$

Therefore, 40 mL of the suspension must be given to the patient in order to administer 2 grams (2,000 mg) of the active ingredient.

Example 9.4

How many milliliters of a 50% dextrose solution should be infused in a patient in order to administer 400 grams of dextrose to the patient?

Solution

A 50% solution of dextrose means that each 100 mL of the solution contains 50 grams of dextrose. In other words, this is what the question is asking: If 100 mL of the solution contains 50 grams of dextrose, how many milliliters will deliver 400 grams of dextrose to the patient?

$$50 \text{ g dextrose} \rightarrow 100 \text{ mL solution}$$

$$400 \text{ g dextrose} \rightarrow u$$

$$u = \frac{100 \text{ mL solution}}{50 \text{ g dextrose}} \times \frac{400 \text{ g dextrose}}{1}$$

$$= 800 \text{ mL solution}$$

Example 9.5

If 400 mL of 10% tannic acid is diluted with distilled water to 1,000 mL, what will be the new percentage strength of the diluted tannic acid?

Solution

We can use our dilution equation here

$$C_1 Q_1 = C_2 Q_2$$

$$10\% \times 400 \text{ mL} = C_2 \times 1,000 \text{ mL}$$

$$C_2 = \frac{10\% \times 400 \text{ mL}}{1,000 \text{ mL}}$$

$$= 4\%$$

Or, alternatively, we can use proportion principles to solve this in two steps:

Step 1. Determine the amount of tannic acid originally in the 400 mL of the 10% solution.

Step 2. Determine the new percentage strength of the tannic acid solution in the new expanded and diluted volume.

Solving for step 1:

A solution of 10% tannic acid means that every 100 mL of the solution contains 10 grams of tannic acid.

$$100 \text{ mL solution} \rightarrow 10 \text{ g tannic acid}$$

$$400 \text{ mL solution} \rightarrow u$$

$$u = \frac{10 \text{ g tannic}}{100 \text{ mL solution}} \times \frac{400 \text{ mL solution}}{1}$$

= 40 g tannic acid contained in the 400 mL solution

Solving for step 2:

Realize that when the tannic acid solution was diluted, only the volume changed (i.e., addition of distilled water increased the volume of the solution while the amount of active ingredient remained the same). The strength of the solution will be reduced (that is, diluted). This step will seek to calculate how many grams of the tannic acid will be in 100 mL of the new diluted solution. The amount of active ingredient in 100 mL of the solution defines the percentage strength.

From previous calculation, it appears that the 40 grams of tannic acid will now find itself in a new volume of 1,000 mL after the dilution. Therefore, we can say that

$$1,000 \text{ mL new solution} \rightarrow 40 \text{ g tannic acid}$$

$$100 \text{ mL new solution} \rightarrow u$$

$$u = \frac{40 \text{ g } tannic}{1{,}000 \text{ mL } solution} \times \frac{100 \text{ mL}}{1}$$

= 4 g of tannic acid in 100 mL of the diluted solution

But percentage strength is defined by the amount of solute in grams contained in 100 mL of the solution. Therefore, the answer "4 g in 100 mL" can also be expressed as 4%.

Example 9.6

A pharmacist accurately weighed out 40 grams of salicylic acid and gave that to the pharmacy technician to prepare a topical 8% salicylic acid ointment by blending the powder with a certain quantity of Vaseline.

(a) What will be the final weight of the correctly compounded ointment if the pharmacy technician used all 40 grams of the salicylic acid?
(b) How many grams of Vaseline will be used in the compounding?

Solution

(a) We can use our dilution equation here. Making of salicylic acid ointment is a kind of dilution where the pure powder (100%) is diluted down to 8%.

$$C_1 Q_1 = C_2 Q_2$$
$$100\% \times 40 \text{ g} = 8\% \times Q_2$$
$$Q_2 = \frac{100\% \times 40 \text{ gram}}{8\%}$$

= 500 g of final formulation

Alternatively, we could use proportion principles.

If the target is to prepare an 8% salicylic acid ointment, it means that every 100 grams of the final ointment must contain 8 grams of salicylic acid as the active ingredient. In effect, this question is asking us how many grams of the formulation can be made using 40 grams of the active ingredient if 8 grams of the active ingredient will give us 100 grams of the formulation.

Using our proportion, we can say

$$8 \text{ g salicylic acid} \rightarrow 100 \text{ g formulation}$$

$$40 \text{ g salicylic acid} \rightarrow u$$

$$u = \frac{100 \text{ g formulation}}{8 \text{ g salicylic acid}} \times \frac{40 \text{ g salicylic acid}}{1}$$

= 500 g of the formulation (ointment)

(b) Ointments are made by adding active ingredient + the inactive base

Ointment = active drug powder + inactive base

500 g = 40 g (pure salicylic acid powder) + Vaseline (inactive base)

500 g – 40 g = Vaseline

Therefore, Vaseline part = 460 g

Or this second part can be solved alternatively using the basic equation that defines the formation of 8% ointment.

8 g salicylic acid + 92 g Vaseline = 100 g
of the formulation (ointment)

From the equation above, it is clear that 92 grams of the Vaseline are needed to make 100 grams of 8% salicylic acid ointment. Then, if 92 grams of Vaseline can make 100 grams of the 8% ointment, how many grams of Vaseline will make 500 grams of the formulation?

Using our principle of the proportion

$$100 \text{ g formulation} \rightarrow 92 \text{ g Vaseline}$$

$$500 \text{ g formulation} \rightarrow u$$

$$u = \frac{92\ g\ vaseline}{100\ g\ formulation} \times \frac{500\ g\ formulation}{1}$$

$$= 460 \text{ g of Vaseline}$$

Therefore, to make 500 grams of the ointment (formulation), we simply need to blend 40 grams of the salicylic acid with 460 grams of the Vaseline.

$$40 \text{ g} + 460 \text{ g} = 500 \text{ g}$$

Example 9.7

How many milliliters of water must be added to 180 mL of 40% stock solution of potassium permanganate in order to reduce the concentration to 10% potassium permanganate solution?

Solution

Here we can use the dilution equation:

$$C_1 Q_1 = C_2 Q_2$$
$$40\% \times 180 \text{ mL} = 10\% \times Q_2$$

$$Q_2 = \frac{40\% \times 180\ mL}{10\%}$$

$$= 720 \text{ mL}$$

So the final volume of the diluted solution will be 720 mL, which means that a certain volume of water (720 mL – 180 mL) must have been added, which is 540 mL.

Alternatively, we can use the proportion principle to solve the problem in three steps.

Step 1. Determine the amount of potassium permanganate present in 180 mL of the 40% stock solution.

Step 2. Determine what volume of solution in which the amount of potassium permanganate calculated in step 1 can exist in order to form a 10% solution.

Step 3. Subtract the final volume from the initial volume to get the amount of vehicle (water) added.

Step 1. A solution of 40% potassium permanganate means that 100 mL of the solution must contain 40 grams of potassium permanganate. If this is so, then how many grams will be found in 180 mL of the solution? This can be solved using our proportion.

That is,

100 mL solution → 40 g potassium permanganate

180 mL solution → u

$$u = \frac{40 \text{ } g \text{ } potassium \text{ } permanganate}{100 \text{ } mL \text{ } solution} \times \frac{180 \text{ } mL \text{ } solution}{1}$$

= 72 g of potassium permanganate present
in the 180 mL of the solution

Step 2. In what volume can 72 grams of potassium permanganate exist in order to produce a 10% solution?

Note: Adding a diluent to an existing solution only changes the concentration but does not change the quantity of active ingredient present in the new diluted solution.

To achieve a 10% solution of potassium permanganate (KMn04), 10 grams of potassium permanganate must be present in 100 mL of the solution. If 10 grams is in 100 mL, 72 grams will be in what volume? Our proportion will quickly answer that.

10 g potassium permanganate → 100 mL solution

72 g potassium permanganate → u

$$u = \frac{100 \text{ mL solution}}{10 \text{ g KmNo4}} \times \frac{72 \text{ g Kmn04}}{1}$$

$$= 720 \text{ mL solution}$$

Step 3. So the initial volume of the solution was 180 mL, and the final volume this time is 720 mL after dilution. Therefore, a certain volume of water must have been added to achieve this, which is

$$720 \text{ mL} - 180 \text{ mL} = 540 \text{ mL of water added.}$$

Example 9.8

How many milliliters of a 1:50 dextrose solution can be made from 250 mL of a 5% dextrose solution?

Solution

Using the dilution equation, we can proceed.

But before we do that, we need to make sure the two concentrations have the same type of expression. Here I will choose to convert the 1:50 ratio strength to percentage.

A ratio of 1:50 means that every 50 mL of the solution contains 1 gram of the dextrose.

$$50 \text{ mL solution} \rightarrow 1 \text{ g dextrose}$$

$$100 \text{ mL solution} \rightarrow u$$

$$u = \frac{1 \text{ g dextrose}}{50 \text{ mL solution}} \times \frac{100 \text{ mL solution}}{1}$$

$$= 2\%$$

$$C_1 Q_1 = C_2 Q_2$$

$$5\% \times 250 \text{ mL} = 2\% \times Q_2$$

$$Q_2 = \frac{5\% \times 250 \text{ mL}}{2\%}$$

$$= 625 \text{ mL}$$

Alternatively, we can use proportion principles in solving.

Interpretation of the question: If you have a 250 mL of dextrose such that every 100 mL contain 5 grams of dextrose and you want to dilute the solution such that every 50 mL of the new diluted solution will now contain 1 gram (1:50), how many milliliters will the dilute solution be?

Again, we can solve this problem using two steps.

Step 1. Determine the amount in grams of dextrose that exists in 250 mL of 5% solution.

Step 2. Find the new volume the solution can be diluted to such that every 50 mL of the new diluted solution will contain only 1 gram of dextrose.

Now solving

Step 1. The given stock solution is a 250 mL 5% dextrose solution. A solution of 5% means that every 100 mL of the solution contains 5 grams of dextrose. If this is so, how many grams of the dextrose will be contained in 250 mL of the solution? Our proportion will lead us to the right answer.

$$100 \text{ mL solution} \rightarrow 5 \text{ g dextrose}$$
$$250 \text{ mL solution} \rightarrow u$$

$$u = \frac{5 \text{ g dextrose}}{100 \text{ mL solution}} \times \frac{250 \text{ mL solution}}{1}$$

$$= 12.5 \text{ g Dextrose}$$

Step 2. Now in what volume shall 12.5 grams of dextrose be dissolved such that every 50 mL of the solution will contain 1 gram of the dextrose (1:50)?

Remember, our target concentration is 1:50, which means each 50 mL of the solution will contain 1 gram of the dextrose. If this is so, how many milliliters will contain the said 12.5 grams of dextrose? Our proportion will be handy in answering this question.

$$1 \text{ g dextrose} \rightarrow 50 \text{ mL solution}$$

$$12.5 \text{ g dextrose} \rightarrow u$$

$$u = \frac{50 \text{ mL solution}}{1 \text{ g dextrose}} \times \frac{12.5 \text{ g dextrose}}{1}$$

$$= 625 \text{ mL}$$

This technically means that 375 mL of water (625 mL – 250 mL) was actually added to the 5% solution in order to reduce the concentration to 1:50.

Example 9.9

An order calls for 250 mL of 8% boric acid, and you have a 40% boric acid solution. How many milliliters of the 40% boric acid will you use?

Solution

We can use the dilution equation.

$$C_1 Q_1 = C_2 Q_2$$

$$40\% \times Q_1 = 8\% \times 250 \text{ mL}$$

$$Q_1 = \frac{8\% \times 250 \text{ mL}}{40\%}$$

$$= 50 \text{ mL}$$

Alternatively, we can solve through proportion principles.

The available strength is 40%. Certain volume of this strength must be diluted to 250 mL in order to get an 8% boric acid solution. To solve this, we again require two steps.

Step 1. Calculate the amount of boric acid in 250 mL of 8% solution (which is the real amount of boric acid actually prescribed). This represents the amount of boric acid desired from the 40% solution.

Step 2. Calculate the volume of the 40% solution that will yield the desired amount of boric acid as calculated in step 1.

Now solving

Step 1. A solution of 8% boric acid means that every 100 mL of the solution contains 8 grams of boric acid. If this is so, how many grams of boric acid will be contained in 250 mL of the same strength of solution? We use our proportion.

$$100 \text{ mL solution} \rightarrow 8 \text{ g boric acid}$$

$$250 \text{ mL solution} \rightarrow u$$

$$u = \frac{8 \text{ g boric acid}}{100 \text{ mL solution}} \times \frac{250 \text{ mL solution}}{1}$$

$$= 20 \text{ g boric acid}$$

Step 2. To obtain 20 grams of boric acid from a 40% solution, we need a certain volume of the solution. A solution of 40% means that every 100 mL of the solution contains 40 grams of the boric acid. If this is so, how many milliliters will contain the 20 grams of boric acid as calculated in step 1? Again, we use our proportion.

$$40 \text{ g boric acid} \rightarrow 100 \text{ mL}$$

$$20 \text{ g boric acid} \rightarrow u$$

$$u = \frac{100 \text{ mL solution}}{40 \text{ g boric acid}} \times \frac{20 \text{ g boric acid}}{1}$$

$$= 50 \text{ mL}$$

Therefore, we need 50 mL of 40% boric acid. We will add extra 200 mL of water to make 250 mL of 8% boric acid solution.

Example 9.10

Approximately 20 mL of dextrose solution was diluted with distilled water to make 120 mL of 8% dextrose solution. What was the original percentage strength of the dextrose solution?

Solution

We use the dilution equation:

$$C_1Q_1 = C_2Q_2$$
$$C_1 \times 20 \text{ mL} = 8\% \times 120 \text{ mL}$$
$$C_1 = \frac{8\% \times 120 \text{ mL}}{20 \text{ mL}}$$
$$= 48\%$$

Alternatively, we can use the proportion principles to solve in two steps.

Step 1. Determine the amount of active ingredient in the 120 mL of the 8% dextrose solution.

Step 2. The answer to step 1 represents the amount of active ingredient that was originally in the 20 mL before the dilution. If this amount of active ingredient was originally in 20 mL, what would be the percentage strength?

Now calculating

Step 1. A solution of 8% means that each 100 mL of the solution contains 8 grams of the active ingredient. If this is so, what amount of the active ingredient will be contained in the 120 mL of the dextrose solution? We use proportion once more.

100 mL → 8 g dextrose

120 mL → u

$$u = \frac{8\ g\ dextrose}{100\ mL} \times \frac{120\ mL}{1}$$

$$= 9.6 \text{ g dextrose}$$

Step 2. This amount of active ingredient (9.6 grams) was originally present in the initial 20 mL before the dilution. We can comfortably say that 9.6 grams of dextrose were contained in 20 mL of the initial solution. If this is correct, how many grams will be in 100 mL of that solution (if the solution can be expanded to 100 mL)? We again use proportion, and the answer will indicate the percentage strength because percentage strength is defined by the amount of active ingredient in grams contained in 100 mL of the solution.

$$20 \text{ mL} \rightarrow 9.6 \text{ g dextrose}$$

$$100 \text{ mL} \rightarrow u$$

$$u = \frac{9.6\ g\ dextrose}{20\ mL} \times \frac{100\ mL}{1}$$

$$= 48 \text{ g dextrose}$$

An amount of 48 grams of dextrose in 100 mL of the solution means 48%.

Chapter 9 Practice Questions

1. A solution contains 40 mg of active ingredient in every 5 mL of solution. Approximately 10 mL of this solution was diluted to 100 mL. What will be the ratio strength of the diluted solution?

2. How many grams of hydrocortisone powder are contained in 5 pounds of a 4% hydrocortisone cream?

3. Approximately 50 grams of dextrose are dissolved in 250 mL of distilled water to form a true solution of dextrose. What is the percentage strength of the solution?

4. You were given 40 grams of diclofenac powder to make an 8% diclofenac ointment in Diffusimax. How many grams of the ointment can you make with the diclofenac provided, assuming you have enough Diffusimax base?

5. You were instructed to make 400 mL of 2% vinegar solution from 10% stock solution available in the pharmacy. How many milliliters of the stock solution will be used?

6. How many milliliters of sterile water should be added to 50 grams of dextrose in order to produce a 2.5% solution?

7. How many milliliters of water must be added to 300 mL of 50% sodium chloride solution in order to prepare a 1.8% sodium chloride solution?

8. You watched a pharmacist pour 800 mL of distilled water into 200 mL of stock solution of sodium bicarbonate. The pharmacist said she has just made a 5% solution. What could possibly be the original percentage concentration of the stock sodium bicarbonate solution?

9. How many milliliters of 4% sodium hypochlorite solution can be prepared from 500 mL of 20% sodium hypochlorite solution?

10. Approximately 30 grams of tannic acid were dissolved in 500 mL of sterile water to form tannic acid solution. What is the percentage strength of the solution?

11. How many grams of adrenaline are contained in 400 mL of 10% adrenaline stock solution?

12. If 20 mL of 1:200 ratio strength of epinephrine is diluted to 100 mL, what will be the percentage strength of the diluted solution?

13. You were provided with 2 grams of sodium hypochlorite powder to make a 0.5% solution in distilled water. What will be the final volume of your solution if you use the entire active ingredient provided?

14. How many milliliters of distilled water must be added to 180 mL of 10% dextrose in order to produce a 4% dextrose solution?

15. If 50 mL of a 1:20 solution of a certain solution is diluted to 2,000 mL, what will be the percentage strength of the resulting solution?

16. You want to make a 3% solution of sucrose in distilled water. In what volume of distilled water should 6 grams of sucrose be dissolved in order to achieve the desired percentage?

17. You receive an order for 200 mL of 5% dextrose. You have a stock of 20% solution of dextrose. How many milliliters of the 20% will you need to make the required volume of the 5% dextrose?

18. A pharmacy technician mistakenly poured 600 mL of distilled water into 400 mL of 10% tannic acid solution. What will be the resulting percentage concentration of the new diluted solution?

19. How many milliliters of a 10 mg/mL solution of tetracycline can be prepared from 50 mL of a 10% solution of tetracycline?

20. A technician dissolved 50 mg of dextrose in 10 mL of distilled water. What will be the ratio strength of the resultant solution?

21. You receive the following prescription:

    Rx
    Sodium bicarbonate solution 1%
        Make 400 mL

    You have in stock a 5% solution of sodium bicarbonate. How many milliliters of the 5% will be used?

22. How many grams of dextrose are contained in 300 mL of a 50% dextrose solution?

23. Approximately 400 mL of 1% iodine solution was diluted to 5,000 mL. What will be the ratio strength of the new dilute solution?

24. A pharmacist weighed out 4 grams of dextrose, and this was given to a pharmacy assistant with the instruction to prepare dextrose solution in distilled water such that every 5 mL of the solution will contain 200 mg of dextrose. What will be the final volume of the preparation?

25. How many milliliters of water should be added to 40 mL of 50% alcohol solution in order to reduce the concentration to 20%?

26. In what volume of sterile water must 75 grams of potassium permanganate be dissolved in order to produce a 15% solution?

27. How many milliliters of sterile water would be added to 50 mL of 8% tannic acid solution in order to produce a 2% solution?

28. You receive the following physician's order:

    Rx
    Epinephrine 1:10,000
        Make 500 mL

    You have in stock a 4% solution of epinephrine.
    How many milliliters of the 4% will you use?

29. A vinegar stock solution of 50 mL was diluted to 250 mL, and the concentration dropped to 1%. What was the original percentage concentration of the stock vinegar solution?

30. You were told to make 0.1% vinegar solution from 0.8% solution. How many milliliters of the 0.1% can be produced from 100 mL of the 0.8% vinegar solution?

31. How many grams of pure diclofenac powder is contained in 500 grams of 8% diclofenac ointment?

32. A pharmacist dissolved 3 grams of sodium bicarbonate in 500 mL of water. How many milligrams of sodium bicarbonate will be contained in every 5 mL of the resulting solution?

33. You were instructed to dilute 500 mL of 8% tetracycline mouthwash to 2 liters. What will be the percentage strength of the new dilute solution?

34. How many milliliters of water must be added to 100 mL of 1% iodine tincture in order to produce a 1:200 tincture of iodine?

35. You have 35 grams of hydrocortisone powder, and you want to make a 2% hydrocortisone cream in Glaxal base. What amount of Glaxal base will be needed to mix with the 35 grams of hydrocortisone in order to produce the 2% hydrocortisone cream?

36. How many milliliters of sterile water for injection must be added to 5 liters of 40% dextrose injection to reduce the concentration to 10%?

37. You have 15 grams of boric acid, and you desire to make a 3% solution. In what volume of water must the 15 grams be dissolved to achieve the desired concentration?

38. A pharmacist diluted 400 mL potassium permanganate to 1.6 L. The new concentration became 1:1,000. What was the original ratio strength of the stock potassium permanganate?

39. You have in stock a 20% boric acid solution. You received an order to prepare a 500 mL of 40 mg/mL solution of boric acid. How many milliliters of the 20% will you use?

40. How many milliliters of 1:1,000 epinephrine solution can be made from 200 mL of 0.5% epinephrine solution?

41. A certain liquid preparation contains 2 grams of the active ingredient in every 200 mL of the preparation. Approximately 800 mL of this preparation was diluted with 200 mL of the neutral vehicle. What will be the resultant ratio strength?

42. How many grams of amino acid are contained in 1 liter of 3% amino acid solution?

43. If 400 mL of 10% boric acid solution is diluted to 1.6 liters, what will be the final percentage strength?

44. You were given 5 grams of dextrose and instructed to make a 0 0.625% solution in distilled water. What will be the final volume of the solution if you used all the active ingredients?

45. A pharmaceutical suspension contains 250 mg of active ingredient in every 5 mL of the suspension. How many milliliters of the vehicle must be added to 200 mL of the solution in order to produce a 1% suspension?

46. If 500 mL of 40% solution is diluted to 4 liters, what will be the resulting percentage strength?

47. How many milliliters of sterile water must be added to 150 mg of sodium bicarbonate in order to make a 15% sodium bicarbonate solution?

48. If 20 tablespoonfuls of a 4% solution are diluted to 1.25 liters, what will be the percentage strength of the resulting diluted solution?

49. Approximately 200 mL of stock solution of boric acid was diluted to 1,000 mL, and the resulting solution now has a concentration of 4%. What could possibly be the original concentration of the stock boric acid solution?

50. How many milliliters of 2.5% solution of potassium permanganate can be prepared from 500 mL of 5% potassium permanganate solution?

★ Star Question ★

In a certain pharmacy, there were 100 mL of phenobarbital suspension labeled 50 mg / 4 mL. The pharmacist accidentally spilled 30 mL of the suspension and then used distilled water to replace the spill to 100 mL and mixed thoroughly. How many milligrams of phenobarbital will be contained in every 4 mL of the new suspension?

Answers to Chapter 9
Practice Questions

1. 1:1,250
2. 90.9 g
3. 20%
4. 500 g
5. 80 mL
6. 2,000 mL
7. 8,033.33 mL
8. 25%
9. 2,500 mL
10. 6%
11. 40 g
12. 0.1%
13. 400 mL
14. 270 mL
15. 0.125%
16. 200 mL
17. 50 mL
18. 4%
19. 500 mL
20. 1:200
21. 80 mL
22. 150 g
23. 1:1,250
24. 100 mL
25. 60 mL
26. 500 mL
27. 150 mL
28. 1.25 mL
29. 5%
30. 800 mL
31. 40 g
32. 30 mg

33. 2%
34. 100 mL
35. 1,715 g
36. 15,000 mL
37. 500 mL
38. 1:250
39. 100 mL
40. 1,000 mL
41. 1:125
42. 30 g
43. 2.5%
44. 800 mL
45. 800 mL
46. 5%
47. 1 mL
48. 0.96%
49. 20%
50. 1,000 mL

Solution to Star Question

Total volume of the phenobarbital suspension was 100 mL. When 30 mL is spilled, the volume remaining will be

$$100 \text{ mL} - 30 \text{ mL} = 70 \text{ mL}$$

The 70 mL remaining contains a certain amount of the active ingredient. It is stated that every 4 mL of the suspension contains 50 mg of phenobarbital.

4 mL suspension → 50 mg phenobarbital

70 mL suspension → u

$$u = \frac{50 \text{ mg phenobarbital}}{4 \text{ mL suspension}} \times \frac{70 \text{ mL suspension}}{1}$$

= 875 mg phenobarbital

So the 70 mL of the remaining suspension contains 875 mg of phenobarbital.

When 30 mL distilled water is added to the 70 mL suspension, the volume becomes

$$70 \text{ mL} + 30 \text{ mL} = 100 \text{ mL}.$$

By adding the distilled water, only the volume changed. The amount of phenobarbital (875 mg) remained unchanged; only concentration changed.

The question wants to know what amount of phenobarbital will be contained in every 4 mL of the new suspension.

We can therefore say

100 mL new → 875 mg phenobarbital

4 mL new → u

$$u = \frac{875 \text{ mg phenobarbital}}{100 \text{ ml new}} \times \frac{4 \text{ mL new}}{1}$$

= 35 mg phenobarbital

The new suspension now contains 35 mg of phenobarbital in every 4 mL of the new suspension. There is clear indication of dilution from 50 mg / 4 mL to 35 mg / 4 mL.

CHAPTER 10

Calculations Involving Intravenous Administration of Fluids and Medications

Objectives

At the end of this chapter, students should be able to do the following:

- Demonstrate understanding of the concept of drop factor
- Solve problems about rate of infusion
- Calculate the infusion time
- Determine volume of infusion

Introduction

At some points in the hospital or home setting, there may be the need to administer medications or fluids via intravenous infusion. Pharmacy professionals wishing to work in the hospital setting must be well-versed in the knowledge and calculations involving intravenous administration of medications and fluids.

Intravenous administration of fluids may be necessary for rehydration or as a means of transporting medications needing rapid distribution, delivery to vital organs, and absorption into the body systems.

Intravenous solutions are usually packaged in 50–1,000 mL containers, mostly in flexible plastic infusion bags (however, some infusion bags have been supplied in sizes outside this range), and each contains both the solute and the solvent according to specific patient needs.

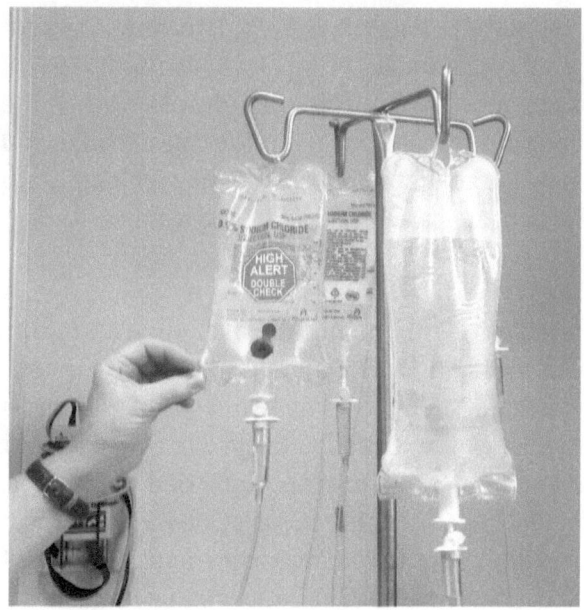

FIGURE 10.1 *The Infusion Bags:* Intravenous solutions are available in 50-1000 mL containers mostly packaged in flexible plastic infusion bags.

Each written prescription of intravenous fluid specifies the following:

- The type of fluid required
- The rate of infusion required
- The volume of fluid to be administered
- If specific medication should be added, the amount and dosage of the medication to be administered

These specifications depend on the nature of the disease being treated, the specific patient condition (disease state, level of dehydration, urgency), and the nature (pharmacology) of the adjunctive medication.

Most solute in intravenous fluid have their concentrations expressed in percentages of solutes in the solution. For example, 10% dextrose solution in water (DW10) means that every 100 mL of the intravenous fluid contains 10 gram of dextrose (10 g / 100 mL).

In this chapter, we will focus on how to determine the rate of flow (in number of drops per minute) of intravenous fluid. We will also focus on how to determine the infusion time/duration when the volume to be infused and the flow rate are given. We can also determine the total time necessary for an amount of fluid to be completely administered as ordered when the rate of infusion and volume to be infused are provided.

However, calculations involving intravenous fluid administration can present some challenges. Students should bear in mind that the calculations are all about the same concept of proportion that has been extensively dealt with and employed in calculations in previous chapters (see chapter 1 for rules of proportion calculations). Just like in other calculations involving medications, extreme care must be exercised in calculations involving intravenous infusions for obvious reasons. The consequence will be catastrophic if a wrong medication, dose, or strength is infused at a wrong rate or involving a wrong volume. When fluids are infused into the vein, it takes nanoseconds to be distributed throughout the body and cannot be retrieved. Therefore, it is absolutely important that the correct solute in a correct volume of a correct fluid be administered at a correct rate and over a correct length of time.

Example 10.1

You receive the prescription of 1,500 mL of 50% dextrose in water (D/W) to be infused into a patient. Calculate the amount of dextrose in grams present in the 1,500 mL of the specified strength of dextrose.

Solution

The solution to this problem begins by understanding what 50% dextrose in water means. It means that every 100 mL of the solution contains 50 grams of dextrose. This forms the basis for our proportional calculations. The question is therefore asking us to determine the amount of dextrose in 1,500 mL of the solution if every 100 mL of the solution contains 50 grams of dextrose.

$$100 \text{ mL solution} \rightarrow 50 \text{ g dextrose}$$

$$1{,}500 \text{ mL solution} \rightarrow u$$

$$u = \frac{50 \ g \ dextrose}{100 \ mL \ solution} \times \frac{1{,}500 \ mL \ solution}{1}$$

$$= 750 \text{ g dextrose}$$

If the patient received the entire 1,500 mL of the D/W, that means 750 grams of dextrose would have been administered to the patient.

Example 10.2

A physician ordered 1,000 mg of an antibiotic to be put into 500 mL of 5% dextrose in water (D-5-W) to be infused into a patient. After the infusion had run for some time, the physician ordered that the infusion be stopped. At the time the infusion was stopped, 200 mL of the infusion was remaining in the infusion bag. Calculate the amount of the antibiotic that had already entered the patient's system when the infusion was discontinued.

Solution

If 200 mL of the infusion was remaining, it means the volume that has entered the patient's system will be

$$500 \text{ mL} - 200 \text{ mL} = 300 \text{ mL}$$

So what amount of the antibiotic was conveyed to the patient's system through the 300 mL infused? The answer again is all about proportion. We know that the entire 1,000 mg of the antibiotic was assumed to be distributed evenly throughout the 500 mL of the intravenous fluid. That is to say that the 500 mL of the intravenous fluid contains 1,000 mg of antibiotic. If this is true, then 300 mL of the intravenous fluid will contain what?

500 mL infusion → 1,000 mg antibiotic

300 mL infusion → u

$$u = \frac{1,000 \; mg \; antibiotic}{500 \; mL \; infusion} \times \frac{300 \; mL \; infusion}{1}$$

= 600 mg antibiotics

Example 10.3

A physician ordered 100 mg of aminophylline to be added to 50 mL of normal saline (NS) for intravenous infusion. You have a 10 mL vial of aminophylline labeled 25 mg/mL.

(a) How many milliliters of the aminophylline solution should be added to the infusion?
(b) If the patient eventually received only 45 mL of the properly constituted intravenous infusion, how many milligrams of aminophylline did the patient receive?

Solution

(a) Aminophylline 25 mg/mL means that each milliliter of the solution contains 25 mg of the active drug. If this is correct, then how many milliliters will fetch us 100 mg of the active medication (aminophylline)? We can apply the concept of proportion to quickly answer this:

25 mg aminophylline → 1 mL solution

100 mg aminophylline → u

$$u = \frac{1 \; mL \; solution}{25 \; mg \; aminophylline} \times \frac{100 \; mg \; aminophylline}{1}$$

= 4 mL aminophylline solution

Therefore adding 4 mL of aminophylline (25 mg/mL) will introduce 100 mg of the pure drug (aminophylline) into the solution as well as increase the volume of the intravenous fluid by 4 mL.

(b) When 4 mL of aminophylline solution is added to the IV bag, the total volume becomes 50 mL + 4 mL = 54 mL.

The 100 mg of aminophylline will be said to be contained in the now 54 mL of the intravenous infusion. 45 mL of this fluid was actually received by the patient. So how many milligrams of aminophylline was contained in the 45 mL?

$$54 \text{ mL IV fluid} \rightarrow 100 \text{ mg aminophylline}$$

$$45 \text{ mL IV fluid} \rightarrow u$$

$$u = \frac{100 \text{ mg aminophylline}}{54 \text{ ml IV fluid}} \times \frac{45 \text{ ml IV fluid}}{1}$$

$$= 83.333 \text{ mg aminophylline}$$

Example 10.4

A physician ordered 250 mg of morphine sulfate to be added to 1 L of 5% dextrose in water. Morphine is available as injectable vials of 12.5 mg / 2.5 mL.

(a) How many milliliters of the morphine solution should be added to the infusion fluid?
(b) If patient only receive 650 mL of the fluid, how many milligrams of the morphine was infused into the patient?
(c) How many grams of dextrose did the patient receive?

Solution

(a) If the morphine is only available as solution containing 12.5 mg of morphine in every 2.5 mL, then how many milliliters will deliver the 250 mg of morphine?

$$12.5 \text{ mg} \rightarrow 2.5 \text{ mL}$$

$$250 \text{ mg} \rightarrow u$$

$$u = \frac{2.5 \ mL}{12.5 \ mg} \times \frac{250 \ mg}{1}$$

= 50 mL of the morphine solution

When this 50 mL of the morphine solution is added to 1 L (1,000 mL) of the intravenous fluid, the total volume will be 1,050 mL.

(b) Now we can say that the 250 mg of morphine will be contained in the 1,050 mL of constituted intravenous fluid. Since only 650 mL was infused, how many milligrams of morphine will be in that 650 mL?

$$1,050 \text{ mL infusion} \rightarrow 250 \text{ mg morphine}$$

$$650 \text{ mL infusion} \rightarrow u$$

$$u = \frac{250 \ mg \ morphine}{1,050 \ mL \ infusion} \times \frac{650 \ mL \ infusion}{1}$$

= 154.76 mg of morphine

(c) A solution of 5% dextrose in water means that every 100 mL of the dextrose solution contains 5 grams of dextrose. If this is so, how many grams of dextrose will be contained in the 1 L of the infusion?

$$100 \text{ mL infusion} \rightarrow 5 \text{ g dextrose}$$

$$1,000 \text{ mL infusion} \rightarrow u$$

$$u = \frac{5 \ g \ dextrose}{100 \ mL \ infusion} \times \frac{1,000 \ mL \ infusion}{1}$$

= 50 g dextrose contained in 1 L of the infusion

When the 50 mL of morphine solution was added to the 1,000 mL (1 L) of the infusion, the amount of dextrose contained in the infusion bag (50 grams) remained unchanged; only the volume of fluid changed to 1,050 mL alongside the concentration of the dextrose in the bag (a decrease in concentration).

Hence, we can say that the new volume of 1,050 mL infusion contains 50 grams of dextrose. If this is true, then how many grams will be contained in the 650 mL of the infusion the patient received?

$$1,050 \text{ mL infusion} \rightarrow 50 \text{ g dextrose}$$
$$650 \text{ mL infusion} \rightarrow u$$

$$u = \frac{50 \text{ g dextrose}}{1,050 \text{ mL infusion}} \times \frac{650 \text{ mL infusion}}{1}$$

= 30.95 g of dextrose received through the 650 mL infusion

Example 10.5

A prescription order instructs that 500 mL of 5% dextrose saline (D-5-S) containing 2 grams of ceftriaxone antibiotic be administered to a patient over eight hours.

(a) Calculate the amount of dextrose contained in the entire infusion bag.
(b) If the complete infusion was set to run for eight hours as ordered but the infusion was stopped at the sixth hour due to some circumstance, consider the following questions.

   (i) How many grams of dextrose would the patient have received?
   (ii) How many milligrams of ceftriaxone would the patient have received?

Solution

(a) A solution of 5% dextrose means that each 100 mL of the solution contains 5 grams of dextrose. Then how many grams of dextrose will be in 500 mL of the solution?

100 mL infusion → 5 g dextrose

500 mL infusion → u

$$u = \frac{5\ g\ dextrose}{100\ mL\ infusion} \times \frac{500\ mL\ infusion}{1}$$

= 25 g of dextrose contained in 500 mL of the infusion

(b) (i) The 25 grams of dextrose in the 500 mL infusion was set to run for eight hours, but the patient only received six hours' worth of dextrose. How many grams of dextrose were delivered to the patient in the said six hours?

8 hours → 25 g dextrose

6 hours → u

$$u = \frac{25\ g\ dextrose}{8\ hours} \times \frac{6\ hours}{1}$$

= 18.75 g dextrose

So the patient received 18.75 grams of dextrose for the said six hours of infusion, and the remaining 6.25 grams (25 – 18.75) were probably wasted in the remainder.

(c) (ii) Similarly, the 2 grams of ceftriaxone antibiotic would have been completely received by the patient if the patient received the infusion for the complete eight hours, but the administration only ran for six hours. We also solve by proportion.

8 hours → 2 g ceftriaxone

6 hours → u

$$u = \frac{2\ g\ ceftriaxone}{8\ hours} \times \frac{6\ hours}{1}$$

= 1.5 g ceftriaxone

The answer to this question was required in milligrams, so we need to convert the 1.5 grams to its milligram equivalent. (See chapter 2, "Interconversion of Units")

$$1 \text{ g} \rightarrow 1{,}000 \text{ mg}$$

$$1.5 \text{ g} \rightarrow \text{u}$$

$$\text{u} = \frac{1{,}000 \text{ mg}}{1 \text{ g}} \times \frac{1.5 \text{ g}}{1}$$

$$= 1{,}500 \text{ mg ceftriaxone}$$

Example 10.6

As a pharmacy technician in a hospital setting, you received the following prescription:

Rx

Cefazolin 50 mg/kg body weight to be added to 500 mL bag of 10% DW

Infuse over 1 hour.

Patient's weight is 88 pounds.

Cefazolin comes as solution in vials labeled 125 mg/mL.

(a) How many milligrams of cefazolin should be added?
(b) How many milliliters of cefazolin solution should be added?
(c) The infusion was set to run for one hour, but if the IV fluid is stopped at 45th minutes, consider the following:

(i) How many milligrams of cefazolin will the patient receive?
(ii) How many milligrams of dextrose will the patient receive?

Solution

(a) Since the dosage is coming per kilogram of the patient's weight, to get the right dosage for the patient, we need to determine the patient's weight in the appropriate unit according to the prescription. The dosage says 50 mg per kg body weight of the patient. We must first of all determine the patient's weight in kilograms. The weight of the patient was provided in pound, so we need to convert this weight to its kilogram equivalent. We know that 2.2 pounds make 1 kg (see chapter 2); therefore, 88 pounds will make how many kilograms?

$$2.2 \text{ pounds} \rightarrow 1 \text{ kg}$$

$$88 \text{ pounds} \rightarrow u$$

$$u = \frac{1 \, kg}{2.2 \, pounds} \times \frac{88 \, pounds}{1}$$

$$= 40 \text{ kg}$$

So the weight of the patient is 88 pounds or 40 kg.

Now the dosage of the cefazolin for the patient is 50 mg/kg. This simply means that for every kilogram weight of the patient, the patient must receive 50 mg of the cefazolin. That is to say that 1 kg weight of the patient will receive 50 mg of cefazolin. If this is the case, what will 40 kg weight of this patient receive?

$$1 \text{ kg body weight} \rightarrow 50 \text{ mg cefazolin}$$

$$40 \text{ kg body weight} \rightarrow u$$

$$u = \frac{50 \, mg \, cefazolin}{1 \, kg} \times \frac{40 \, kg}{1}$$

$$= 2{,}000 \text{ mg cefazolin}$$

This patient must be set up to receive 2,000 mg of cefazolin in one hour through the intravenous fluid. Therefore, 2,000 mg of cefazolin must be added to the infusion bag and infused into the patient over one hour, according to the prescription.

(b) The cefazolin is not available as pure powder that can simply be weighed and poured into the IV bag. Rather, it is available as a solution containing 125 mg cefazolin in every 1 mL of the solution. Hence, certain volume of that solution will give us the desired 2,000 mg of the pure drug.

$$125 \text{ mg} \rightarrow 1 \text{ mL}$$

$$2{,}000 \text{ mg} \rightarrow u$$

$$u = \frac{1 \text{ } mL}{125 \text{ } mg} \times \frac{2{,}000 \text{ } mg}{1}$$

=16 mL of the cefazolin solution

We need to add 16 mL of the cefazolin solution to the infusion bag in order to be sure we have 2,000 mg of cefazolin in the bag for intravenous administration.

(c)

(i) Running the full content of the bag for one hour (sixty mins) will deliver all the cefazolin (2,000 mg) to the patient. But in this case, the infusion was aborted at the forty-fifth minute of the infusion, which means the patient only received a portion of the cefazolin.

$$60 \text{ mins} \rightarrow 2{,}000 \text{ mg cefazolin}$$

$$45 \text{ mins} \rightarrow u$$

$$u = \frac{2{,}000 \text{ } g \text{ } cefazolin}{60 \text{ } min} \times \frac{45 \text{ } min}{1}$$

= 1,500 mg cefazolin

(**Note:** the two indicators of time (hour and minute) must be interconverted to one unit, either in min or in hour, for the calculation to proceed correctly.)

(ii) Similarly, 10% dextrose water means that every 100 mL of the solution contains 10 grams of dextrose. So how many grams of dextrose will be contained in the 500 mL DW?

100 mL solution → 10 g dextrose

500 mL solution → u

$$u = \frac{10 \ g \ dextrose}{100 \ mL \ solution} \times \frac{500 \ mL \ solution}{1}$$

= 50 g dextrose

The 50 grams of dextrose were scheduled to be administered in one hour of infusion, but the procedure was aborted in the forty-fifth minute. We can calculate the amount of dextrose received by the patient within the forty-five minutes using the concept of proportion.

60 minutes → 50 g dextrose

45 minutes → u

$$u = \frac{50 \ g \ dextrose}{60 \ min} \times \frac{45 \ min}{1}$$

= 37.5 g dextrose

Example 10.7

A physician ordered that 100 mg of aminophylline be added to 1 L of normal saline (NS) and the intravenous fluid infused into a patient for four hours. Aminophylline is available as an injectable solution labeled 25 mg/mL.

(a) How many milliliters of the aminophylline should be added to the 1 L of the NS?
(b) How many milligrams of aminophylline will be present per milliliter of the IV normal saline?
(c) How many milligrams of aminophylline would have been infused into the patient at 50 minutes and at 1.5 hours?

Solution

(a) Each milliliter of the aminophylline solution contains 25 mg of aminophylline active ingredient. If this is true, then how many

milliliters will deliver 100 mg of aminophylline to the IV bag?
We again use proportion.

25 mg aminophylline → 1 mL solution

100 mg aminophylline → u

$$u = \frac{1 \; mL \; solution}{25 \; mg \; aminophylline} \times \frac{100 \; mg \; of \; aminophylline}{1}$$

= 4 mL of the aminophylline solution

Therefore, by the addition of 4 mL of the aminophylline
solution (25 mg/5mL), 100 mg of the aminophylline pure drug
will be added to the intravenous fluid.

(b) When the 4 mL of the aminophylline solution is added to 1 L
(1,000 mL) of the normal saline, the volume of the mixture
changes to

1,000 mL + 4 mL = 1,004 mL

Now remember that the 100 mg of the aminophylline will
be uniformly distributed throughout the 1,004 mL of fluid
in the infusion bag. We can therefore say that 100 mg of
aminophylline is contained in 1,004 mL of the solution. If this
is true, how many milligrams of the aminophylline will be
contained in each milliliter of the mixture?

1,004 mL mixture → 100 mg aminophylline

1 mL mixture → u

$$u = \frac{100 \; mg \; aminophylline}{1,004 \; mL \; mixture} \times \frac{1 \; mL}{1}$$

=0.0996 mg in every 1 mL of the IV fluid.

(c) If the infusion was originally set to run for four hours, it means
that the entire 100 mg of aminophylline would be set to be
completely infused in four hours. If this is true, then how
much of the aminophylline will enter the patient's system in

fifty minutes? Realize that four hours is equivalent to 4 × 60 minutes = 240 mins. Using our proportion, we can say that

240 mins → 100 mg aminophylline

50 mins → u

$$u = \frac{100 \; mg \; aminophylline}{240 \; mins} \times \frac{50 \; mins}{1}$$

= 20.833 mg of aminophylline

Similarly at 1.5 hours (which is 90 minutes), we can also calculate the amount of aminophylline in milligrams already infused into the patient's body. Thus

240 mins → 100 mg aminophylline

90 mins → u

$$u = \frac{100 \; mg \; aminophylline}{240 \; mins} \times \frac{90 \; mins}{1}$$

= 37.5 mg aminophylline

Calculations Involving Flow Rates — Some Special Notes

In some instances, fluids may be infused without any added medications. Conversely, in other situations, intravenous fluids may have some medications added into it for therapeutic reasons. The rate at which the medication may be administered to the patient varies depending on the nature of the fluid or the medication it contains and the specific condition of the patient. In most instances, the order from the prescriber may include the following:

- The number of milliliters per unit time to be administered
- The length of time in which the infusion should be administered

In both circumstances, we will be required to determine the number of drops or milliliters that will be discharged from the infusion tubing per minute. This is called the flow rate.

The flow rate of infusion fluid is the function of its drop factor. The drop factor is the number of drops of a fluid from particular tubing that makes up one milliliter. For example, if it takes 60 drops from a tubing to make up 1 mL, then the drop factor is 60.

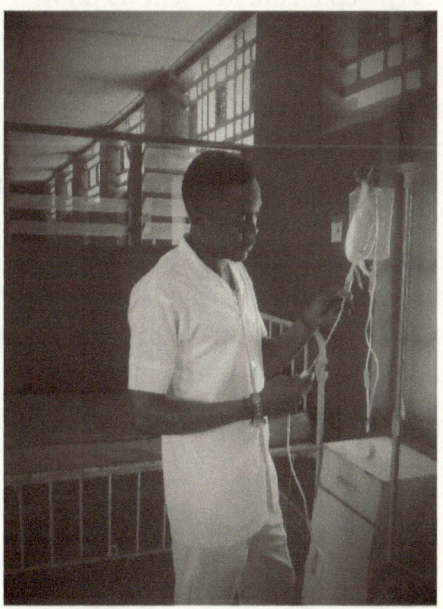

FIGURE 10.2 *Flow Rate Adjustment:* The rate of flow (drops per minute) of infusions can be manually controlled by adjusting the flow regulator of the roller clamp, counting the number of drops while timing with a stop watch

It should be noted that the drop factor of a particular tubing is determined by some factors such as the following:

- *The diameter of the tubing.* The wider the diameter of the tubing, the bigger the size of a drop and the fewer the number of drops that can make up one milliliter, hence the smaller the drop factor.
- *The design of the drop orifice.* The orifice of the dropper can be designed to either enhance flow or restrict flow. When the orifice of a dropper is designed to restrict the flow of a fluid, it means the size of each drop will be less and more drops will be needed to make up 1 mL, thus a higher drop factor, and vice versa.

- *The viscosity of the fluid.* This is one of the factors external to the tubing that can affect the drop factor. A viscous fluid will likely produce a larger drop. This means that few drops of a viscous fluid from the tubing will be more likely to make up 1 mL, thus the consequence will be a lower drop factor, and vice versa.

A higher drop factor means that more number of drops of the fluid from the said tubing will make up 1 mL. A lower drop factor means that a fewer number of drops of a fluid from the said tubing will make up 1 mL.

The knowledge and application of drop factor is very essential in flow rate calculations. Most manufacturers provide the drop factor of the infusion tubing, and this enables the health-care provider to perform some necessary calculations surrounding flow rate.

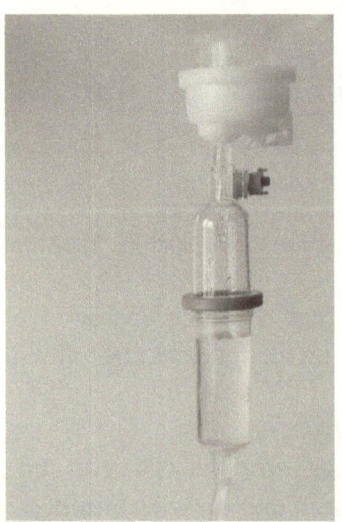

FIGURE 10.3 *The Drip Chamber:* In this chamber, the number of drops per minute can be counted. The drop factor of the infusion set determines the number of drops that can make 1 mL. The lower the drop factor, the larger the size of individual drops (less number of drops per mL) and the higher the drop factor, the smaller the size of each individual drop (more number of drops per mL).

If the drop factor of infusion tubing is 40, it means that 40 drops of fluid from the tubing will be enough to make 1 mL. This information can be represented proportionally, thus

40 drops → 1 mL

or

1 mL → 40 drops

With these lines of proportion, we should be able to calculate the number of drops possible for a given volume of fluid. We should also be able to calculate the volume equivalent to a given number of drops.

For example, if the drop factor of infusion tubing is 40 and the liquid in the infusion bag is 250 mL, how many drops will the infusion set deliver?

From the drop factor of 40, we know that 1 mL is equivalent to 40 drops. Using proportion, we can complete our puzzle.

1 mL → 40 drops

250 mL → u

$$u = \frac{40 \; drops}{1 \; mL} \times \frac{250 \; mL}{1}$$

= 10,000 drops of the fluid

If the physician wants a nurse to administer 120 drops of infusion fluid every minute to a patient, how many milliliters should that represent if the drop factor is 30?

A drop factor of 30 means that each milliliter will deliver 30 drops of the fluid from the infusion set.

$$30 \text{ drops} \rightarrow 1 \text{ mL}$$

$$120 \text{ drops} \rightarrow u$$

$$u = \frac{1 \text{ mL}}{30 \text{ drops}} \times \frac{120 \text{ drops}}{1}$$

$$= 4 \text{ mL}$$

In other words, the physician is actually instructing that 4 mL be administered to the patient per minute (as long as the infusion set with a drop factor of 30 is used).

We use tubing with a low drop factor (fewer drops are needed to make 1 mL) when fluids must be administered at a rapid rate or when a large volume of fluid must be administered at a very short time. Conversely, we use tubing with a high drop factor (many drops are needed to make 1 mL) for a slower delivery of fluids or when small volumes of fluid are to be administered at a very slow rate.

The physician's order is only complete when the total volume of fluid to be administered (milliliter), the rate of flow of the fluid (drops per minutes), and the time for the fluid to infuse (minutes) are well established. All these variables are indirectly governed by the drop factor of the infusion tubing. When two of the variables are known, the remaining can easily be calculated, as we can see from the following examples.

Example 10.8

The physician ordered that 2 L of normal saline be infused into a dehydrated patient over 6 hours. The infusion administration set reads 18 drops/mL (this is the drop factor). At what rate (drops per minute) should the infusion be set?

Solution

The solution to this can be achieved in two simple steps. In solving rate problems, we must realize that we should work with volumes in milliliters and the time in minutes because our answer must be in drops per minute.

$$2 \text{ L is equivalent to } 2 \times 1,000 \text{ mL} = 2,000 \text{ mL}$$

$$6 \text{ hrs} = 6 \times 60 \text{ mins} = 360 \text{ mins}$$

Step 1. Calculate the volume of the infusion that must be infused per minute.

The prescription order requires 2 L (2,000 mL) to be infused over 6 hours (360 mins).

That is to say,

$$360 \text{ mins} \rightarrow 2,000 \text{ mL}$$

$$1 \text{ min} \rightarrow u$$

$$u = \frac{2,000 \ ml}{360 \ mins} \times \frac{1 \ min}{1}$$

$$= 5.55556 \text{ mL per minute}$$

So the rate of delivery must be 5.55556 mL per minute, which means that 5.5556 mL of the infusion must be delivered to the patient in every minute in order for 2,000 mL to be completely delivered to the patient in 6 hours.

Step 2. Convert the milliliters to its drop equivalent using the drop factor.

The question we are asking here is this: How many drops does the 5.5556 mL represent, considering the drop factor?

The drop factor of 18 drops/mL means that each milliliter of the fluid is equivalent to 18 drops. That is,

$$1 \text{ mL} \rightarrow 18 \text{ drops}$$

$$5.5556 \text{ mL} \rightarrow u$$

$$u = \frac{18 \ drops}{1 \ mL} \times \frac{5.5556 \ mL}{1}$$

$$= 100 \text{ drops}$$

So 5.5556 mL is technically equivalent to 100 drops

So the rate will be 5.55556 mL per min or *100 drops* per minute. So the infusion must be set at 100 drops per minute.

Example 10.9

A physician ordered 1.5 L of 5% dextrose saline to be infused into a lethargic patient over 8 hours in the hospital setting. At what rate (drop per minute) should the infusion be set to achieve this target if the drop factor of the infusion set is 16 gtt/mL?

Solution

Calculate the volume of the infusion that must be infused into the patient per minute in order for the entire fluid to be completely administered in 8 hours.

$$1.5 \text{ L} = 1.5 \times 1{,}000 \text{ mL} = 1{,}500 \text{ mL}$$

$$8 \text{ hour} = 8 \times 60 \text{ min} = 480 \text{ min}$$

$$480 \text{ min} \rightarrow 1{,}500 \text{ mL}$$

$$1 \text{ min} \rightarrow u$$

$$u = \frac{1{,}500 \text{ ml}}{480 \text{ min}} \times \frac{1 \text{ min}}{1}$$

$$= 3.125 \text{ mL in 1 min} = 3.125 \text{ mL/min}$$

Therefore, 3.125 mL must be delivered to the patient in 1 minute for the entire 1.5 L to be completely delivered to the patient in 8 hours.

But we are interested in the number of drops per minute, not the volume per minute. We need to convert the volume of 3.125 mL to its drop equivalent, being guided by the drop factor.

$$1 \text{ mL} \rightarrow 16 \text{ drops}$$

$$3.125 \text{ mL} \rightarrow u$$

$$u = \frac{16 \; drops}{1 \; mL} \times \frac{3.125 \; mL}{1}$$

$$= 50 \; drops$$

Therefore, 3.125 mL is equivalent to 50 drops. Hence, 3.125 mL/min also means 50 drops per min.

So the infusion must be set to 50 drops per minute in order to fully administer 1.5 liters of the fluid over 8 hours.

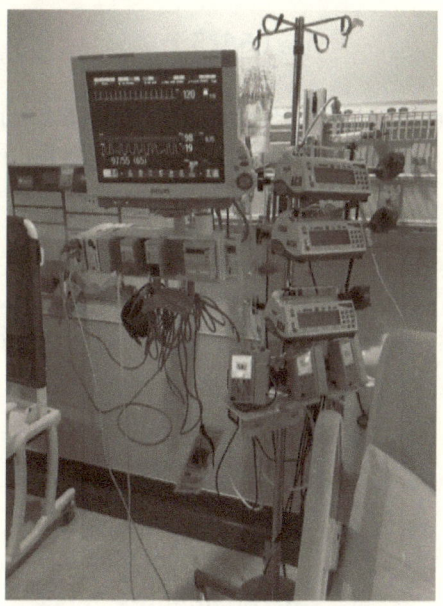

FIGURE 10.4 *Infusion Administration in a Technologically Advanced Hospital:* This can be far from simplified. Sophisticated machines could be a component and the flow rate of the infusion is usually controlled by simple machines manipulated by humans.

Example 10.10

A certain prescription order requires that 2 L of Ringer's lactate be infused into a patient at the rate of 25 drops per minute. The drop factor of the infusion set is 16 drops/mL. How long will it take for the infusion to be completely administered to the patient?

Solution

Step 1. The rate of flow is prescribed to be 25 drops per minute. The question is, how many milliliters do the 25 drops represent? We can get the answer using proportion that employs the drop factor.

$$16 \text{ drops} \rightarrow 1 \text{ mL}$$

$$25 \text{ drops} \rightarrow u$$

$$u = \frac{1\ mL}{16\ drops} \times \frac{25\ drops}{1}$$

$$= 1.5625 \text{ mL}$$

Therefore, 25 drops is equivalent to 1.5625 mL, and 25 drops per minute is the same as 1.5625 mL per minute (as far as the drop factor of 16 is true).

Step 2. Calculate the length of time it will take the 2 L to be infused into the patient if 1.5625 mL is delivered to the patient every minute. Realize that 2 L is equivalent to 2 × 1,000 mL = 2,000 mL.

$$1.5625 \text{ mL} \rightarrow 1 \text{ min}$$

$$2,000 \text{ mL} \rightarrow u$$

$$u = \frac{1\ min}{1.5625\ mL} \times \frac{2,000\ mL}{1}$$

$$= 1,280 \text{ minutes}$$

This value of time can be converted to hours if need be, thus

$$60 \text{ min} \rightarrow 1 \text{ hour}$$

$$1,280 \text{ min} \rightarrow u$$

$$u = \frac{1\ hour}{60\ min} \times \frac{1,280\ min}{1}$$

$$= 21.33 \text{ hours.}$$

So it will take 21.33 hours for the entire 2 L infusion to be delivered to the patient at the rate of 25 drops per minute (1.5625 mL/min).

Exercise 10.11

A physician ordered that a patient be infused with 5% dextrose water at the rate of 24 drops per minute for 12 hours. The drop factor is 15 drops/mL. What volume of the 5% dextrose water will be administered to the patient for that recommended length of time and at that rate?

Solution

By "24 drops per minute," it means that 24 drops of the fluid is delivered to the patient every 1 minute. If this is true, then how many drops of the fluid will be delivered to the patient in 12 hours? Realize that 12 hours is (12 × 60 mins =) 720 mins.

$$1 \text{ min} \rightarrow 24 \text{ drops}$$
$$720 \text{ min} \rightarrow u$$

$$u = \frac{24 \text{ drops}}{1 \text{ min}} \times \frac{720 \text{ min}}{1}$$

$$= 17{,}280 \text{ drops for the total of 12 hours}$$

But what does this number of drops mean in terms of volume? The drop factor will guide us to calculate that.

A drop factor of 15 drops per milliliter means that every 15 drops of the fluid from the said infusion set is equivalent to 1 mL. If this is correct, then what volume will be equivalent to 17,280 drops?

$$15 \text{ drops} \rightarrow 1 \text{ mL}$$
$$17{,}280 \text{ drops} \rightarrow u$$

$$u = \frac{1 \text{ mL}}{15 \text{ drops}} \times \frac{17{,}280 \text{ drops}}{1}$$

$$= 1{,}152 \text{ mL, or approximately } 1{,}150 \text{ mL}$$

Chapter 10 Practice Questions

1. You receive a prescription of 250 mL of 5% dextrose to be infused into the patient over 8 hours. What amount of dextrose (in grams) will the patient receive after the complete infusion of 250 mL?

2. A pharmacist with Additional Prescribing Authorization ordered 500 mL of 10% dextrose in water to be infused into a patient over 6 hours. However, the patient could only receive the infusion for 90 minutes when the infusion was stopped due to unforeseen circumstances.

   (a) What volume of the infusion was administered?
   (b) What amount of dextrose did the patient receive?

3. You received an order requiring 750 mg of an antibiotic to be mixed in 1 L infusion. The patient only received 250 mL of the infusion. What amount of the antibiotics in milligrams was received by the patient?

4. A consultant in pain management ordered that 200 mg of morphine be added to 1 L of lactated ringer's solution and infused into the patient. Morphine is available in the hospital dispensary as an injectable solution labeled as 10 mg / 5 mL.

   (a) How many milliliters of morphine solution should be added to the infusion bag?
   (b) How many milligrams of morphine will be present in every 5 mL of the infusion fluid?
   (c) If the patient received only 300 mL of the infusion fluid, what amount of morphine in milligrams did the patient receive?

5. An amount of 2 L of 3% dextrose was scheduled to be administered to the patient as intravenous infusion over 8 hours.

   (a) If the entire volume of the fluid was administered, how many grams of dextrose would the patient receive?
   (b) If the infusion was stopped at 2 hours 15 minutes, what volume of the fluid would have been administered to the patient?
   (c) If only 1.5 L of the intravenous fluid was administered to the patient, what amount of dextrose would the patient have received?

6. An antihypertensive was prescribed as 10 mg/kg body weight of the patient. The appropriate dose of the antihypertensive is to be added to 500 mL of 5% dextrose water for infusion over 4 hours. The patient weighs 30 kg.

   (a) How many milligrams of the antihypertensive should be the dosage for the patient?
   (b) If the antihypertension is available as injectable solution labeled as 5 mg/mL, how many milliliters of the solution should be added to the intravenous fluid?

7. A physician ordered that 500 mL of normal saline be infused into a patient over 8 hours. The infusion administration set has a drop factor of 15 drops/mL. At what rate (drops per minute) should the infusion be set in order to achieve delivering the entire 500 mL over 8 hours?

8. A physician ordered 1.5 L of normal saline containing 800 mg of an antibiotic to be infused into a patient at the rate of 20 drops per minute. The drop factor of the infusion set is 16 (16 drops per milliliter). How long will it take for the patient to receive the entire volume of the infusion?

9. A physician ordered that a patient be infused with normal saline at the rate of 23 drops per minute for 8 hours. The drop factor of the administrating infusion set is 10 drops per milliliter. What volume of the intravenous fluid is the patient likely to receive?

10. A physician ordered 500 mL of 10% dextrose water to be infused into a patient. Calculate the amount of dextrose in grams present in the entire volume to be infused.

11. A physician orders a continuous infusion of 1,000 mL of 10% dextrose containing 80 mEq of KCl for 12 hours.

   (a) What amount of KCl (in milliequivalents) will be contained in each 50 mL of the infusion fluid?
   (b) How many milliequivalents of KCl will the patient receive each hour through the IV fluid, according to the prescription?
   (c) How many milligrams of dextrose should the patient receive every minute, according to the prescription?

12. A 2 L intravenous fluid containing 1 gram of ceftriaxone antibiotic was meant to be infused into a patient over 8 hours. The patient could not tolerate the side effects of ceftriaxone, and the infusion was stopped at 2 hours 15 minutes.

   (a) What amount of ceftriaxone did the patient receive?
   (b) What volume of intravenous fluid was administered to the patient?

13. You receive an order for 500 mL of normal saline to be infused into a patient over 10 hours. For this infusion to last the desired length of time, consider these questions:

   (a) How many milliliters of the infusion should the patient receive per hour?

(b) How many milliliters of the infusion should the patient receive per minute?

(c) If the drop factor is 15 (15 drops per milliliter), how many drops of the fluid should the patient receive per minute?

14. A general practitioner ordered that 2 grams of an antibiotic be poured into 2 L of 10% dextrose water and infused into the patient over 12 hours. The antibiotic is available as a power whose proper reconstitution will yield a suspension containing 20 mg of the antibiotics in every 5 mL of the suspension.

(a) How many milliliters of the antibiotic suspension will be added?

(b) How many milligrams of the antibiotics will be contained in every 50 mL of the infusion fluid?

(c) If the patient received only 1.5 L of the infusion, how many milligrams of the antibiotics did the patient receive?

15. A 500 mL intravenous fluid bag of 10% dextrose in water containing 200 mg of antibiotic was scheduled to be infused into a patient over 8 hours.

(a) If the entire volume of the IV fluid was administered, what amount of dextrose in grams will the patient receive?

(b) If the infusion was stopped at 2 hours, what amount of the antibiotics would the patient receive?

(c) If only 180 mL of the infusion was administered, how long did that take?

16. An antiemetic was prescribed as 4 mg/kg to be added to 1 L of 10% dextrose saline for infusion over 8 hours to a nauseated patient. Patient weighs 88 pounds.

(a) What amount of the antiemetic will constitute the appropriate dosage for the patient?

(b) If only 300 mL of the infusion was administered to the patient, approximately how many milligrams of the antiemetic did the patient receive?

17. You receive the following prescription:

Rx

Lactated Ringer's solution

Infuse @ rate of 25 drops per min for 10 hours

How many milliliters of the solution is the patient likely to receive in the prescribed 10 hours if the drop factor of the infusion set is 16 drops per milliliter?

18. Approximately 1.5 liters of Ringer's lactate containing 100 mg of antibiotics were ordered to be infused into a patient over 10 hours. The drop factor for the infusion set is 16 drops per milliliter. What will be the rate of administration (drops/min) at which the infusion must be set?

19. You receive the following prescription:

Rx

10% dextrose water 500 mL

for IV infusion @25 drops/min

Drop factor of the infusion set is 15 drops/mL.

How long will it take for the entire fluid to be administered to the patient at the prescribed rate?

20. You received an order of 2,000 mL of 10% dextrose water to be infused into a patient over 12 hours. The drop factor of the infusion set is 20 drops per milliliters.

(a) How many milliliters should the patient receive per hour?

(b) How many milliliters should the patient receive per minute?

(c) How many drops should the patient receive per minute?

21. A physician ordered 2 L of 0.45% NaCl solution to be infused into the patient over 8 hours. If the patient receives the entire 2 L, what amount of NaCl in grams has the patient received?

22. Approximately 100 mg of hydrocortisone was mixed in 2 L of Ringer's lactate for infusion into a patient. The infusion was stopped when only 1.35 L of the infusion was remaining in the infusion bag. What amount of hydrocortisone did the patient receive?

23. A physician ordered that 200 mg of aminophylline be added to 50 mL of D-5-W and infused into the patient over 5 hours. The infusion line was stopped after 30 minutes due to the patient's complaints of palpitation.

(a) What volume of the infusion was administered?

(b) What amount of dextrose was administered?

(c) What amount of aminophylline was administered?

24. A physician ordered 80 mg of KCl to be added to 500 mL of 5% dextrose water and then the mixture to be infused into a hypokalemic patient over 4 hours.

(a) If the entire volume of the intravenous fluid is infused, what amount of dextrose did the patient receive?

(b) Approximately what amount of KCl will be contained in every 10 mL of the infusion fluid?

(c) If only 200 mL of the intravenous fluid was administered to the patient, what amount of the KCl would the patient receive?

(d) If the administration was stopped after 1 hour, what amount of dextrose in grams would the patient have received?

25. A physician ordered that 2,000 mg of ceftriaxone antibiotic be added to 500 mL of 0.45% NaCl solution for intravenous administration. The ceftriaxone antibiotic is available as injectable solution containing 50 mg/mL.

(a) How many milliliters of the antibiotic solution should be added to the infusion bag?

(b) How many milligrams of the ceftriaxone will be contained in 10 mL of the intravenous fluid mixture?

(c) How many milligrams of NaCl will be present in the entire intravenous fluid?

26. The dosage of an antihypertensive medication is 150 mg/kg body weight of the patient. The appropriate dosage must be added to 500 mL of normal saline for infusion into the patient over 8 hours. The patient weighs 100 pounds, and the antihypertensive comes as an injectable solution labeled 3 mg/mL.

(a) How many milligrams of the antihypertensive should be added to the infusion bag?

(b) How many milliliters of the antihypertensive injectable solution should be added to the intravenous fluid bag?

(c) If only 250 mL of the infusion is administered, how many milligrams of the antihypertensive did the patient receive?

27. A physician ordered that 1 L of 5% dextrose saline be infused into a patient over 10 hours. The drop factor for the infusion set is 20 drops/mL. What will be the rate at which the infusion must be set (drops per minute)?

28. You receive the following prescription:

Rx

Dextrose 10% in water

Infuse at rate of 30 drops/min for 6 hours.

———

How many milliliters of the infusion is the patient likely to receive at the end of 6 hours if the drop factor of the infusion set is 20 drops per milliliter?

29. You receive an order to infuse 500 mL of 50% dextrose in water into a patient who was suffering from hypoglycemia. How many grams of dextrose will be delivered to the patient by the 500 mL solution?

30. A physician requested that 2 L of lactated Ringer's solution containing 80 mEq of potassium chloride be infused into a hypokalemic patient at a slow rate of 10 drops per min. The drop factor of the administration set is 16 (16 drops/mL). How long will it take for the patient to receive the entire fluid?

31. A physician orders a 2 L of 10% dextrose water for infusion into a patient over 8 hours. The drop factor for the infusion set is 16 (16 drops per milliliter).

    (a) What is the amount (in grams) of dextrose in 250 mL of the infusion fluid?
    (b) What is the amount (in grams) of dextrose in the entire intravenous fluid?
    (c) How many milliliters of the intravenous fluid should be administered to the patient in 2 hours, according to the prescription?
    (d) How many milliliters of the intravenous fluid should be administered to the patient per minute, according to the prescription?
    (e) At what rate (drops per minute) should the fluid be administered, according to the prescription?

32. A 1 L infusion of 5% dextrose in water contains 20 mEq of potassium chloride. The patient only receives 750 mL of this infusion before the line was disconnected.

(a) What amount of dextrose was administered to the patient?

(b) What amount of potassium chloride in mEq was received by the patient?

33. A 1 liter bag of 10% dextrose saline contains 300 mg of a beta blocker. The intravenous fluid was set to be infused over 5 hours into a patient.

   (a) How many grams of dextrose are contained in the intravenous fluid bag?

   (b) What is the percentage concentration of the beta blocker in the intravenous fluid bag?

   (c) If the patient received the intravenous fluid for only 45 minutes and the line was stopped, what amount of the beta blocker would the patient have received?

34. A consultant ordered that 1 L of 10% dextrose in water containing 200 mg of morphine be infused into a patient over 12 hours. The patient experienced severe respiratory depression at 3.75 hours, and the infusion had to be stopped.

   (a) What volume of the infusion was administered to the patient?

   (b) What amount of dextrose did the patient receive?

   (c) What amount of morphine did the patient receive?

35. The dosage of a narcotic analgesic is 25 mg/kg of the patient weight and is prescribed to add the appropriate dosage to 1 L of 10% dextrose saline and infused into the patient over 4 hours. The patient weighs 70 kg. The narcotic comes as vials of injectable solution labeled as 5 mg / 3mL.

   (a) How many milligrams of the narcotic is the dosage for the patient, according to the prescription?

   (b) How many milliliters of the narcotic injectable solution must be added to the intravenous fluid bag?

(c) What amount of the narcotic will be contained in every 10 mL of the infusion fluid mixture?

(d) If only 450 mL of the infusion was given, how many milligrams of dextrose would the patient receive?

36. A geriatric consultant ordered that 4.8 million units of penicillin Vk antibiotics be added in 2 L of 10% dextrose water. You have available in the dispensary vials of penicillin k solution labeled 5,000 units/mL.

(a) How many milligrams of the penicillin k solution should be added to the infusion fluid?

(b) If only 800 mL of the infusion was infused into the patient, how many units of the antibiotic did the patient receive?

(c) If only 800 mL of the infusion was administered to the patient, what amount of dextrose in grams was received by the patient?

37. Approximately 10 mL of aminophylline injection solution labeled 25 mg / 5mL was mixed with 500 mL of normal saline, and the resulting mixture is to be infused into a patient over 12 hours. The drop factor for the infusion set is 16 (16 drops/mL).

(a) What will be the volume administered per minute to the patient?

(b) How many drops will be administered per minute to the patient?

38. A physician ordered that a continuous infusion of 10% dextrose saline containing 800 mg of morphine be infused into the patient for 8 hours at the rate of 15 drops per min. What is the volume of fluid the patient will receive in the entire 8 hours if the drop factor of the infusion set is 20 drops per milliliter?

39. A physician ordered that 500 mL of 5% dextrose water and 1.5 L of normal saline be mixed and administered to a dehydrated geriatric patient at the rate of 75 drops per minute. (The drop factor for the administration set is 20 drops/mL.) If the patient started receiving the infusion at the prescribed rate by 10 a.m., when is the patient likely going to finish the infusion?

40. A medication used in the treatment of duodenal ulcer has the dosage of 40 mg/kg of patient weight. A required amount of this medication must be added to 500 mL of lactated Ringer's solution and infused into a patient over 12 hours. The patient weighs 105.6 pounds, and the medication comes as an injectable solution labeled 5 mg / 2 mL.

   (a) How many milligrams of medication should be added to the infusion bag?
   (b) How many milliliters of the injectable solution must be added to the infusion bag?
   (c) What is the percentage concentration of the medication in the infusion bag?
   (d) If the infusion was administered for only 1 hour 25 minutes, how many milligrams of the medication did the patient receive?

41. A physician ordered that a patient be infused 0.5 L of normal saline containing 1,500 units of insulin. However, the patient experienced signs of hypoglycemia, and the line was disconnected when the patient received only 200 mL of the infusion. What amount of insulin was administered to the patient?

42. A physician ordered 250 mg of an anti-infective to be mixed in 2 L of 5% dextrose saline and infused into a patient over 12 hours. The drop factor of the administration set is 20 drops per milliliter.

(a) How many milliliters of the infusion fluid should the patient receive in 1 hour?

(b) How many milliliters of the fluid should the patient receive per minute?

(c) How many drops of the fluid should the patient receive per minute?

(d) What is the ratio strength of the anti-infective in the intravenous fluid?

(e) How many milligrams of the anti-infective are present in every milliliter of the infusion solution?

(f) What amount of the anti-infective (in micrograms) will be delivered by each drop of the infusion solution?

43. A physician wants 1 L of 3% dextrose saline to be infused into a patient. If the patient received the entire 1 L, what amount of dextrose has the patient received?

44. Approximately 500 mg of ceftazidime is contained in 2 L of 10% dextrose saline, and the intravenous fluid was set to be administered to a patient as infusion over 6 hours.

(a) How many milligrams of the ceftazidime are contained in 10 mL of the infusion fluid?

(b) How many milligrams of dextrose are contained in every 10 mL of the infusion fluid?

(c) If only 850 mL of the infusion was administered to the patient, how many milligrams of ceftazidime would the patient have received?

45. Approximately 200 mg of Lasix was ordered to be added to 500 mL of dextrose 5% in water and infused into the patient. Lasix is available as an injectable solution labeled 50 mg / 2 mL.

(a) How many milliliters of the Lasix solution should be added to the infusion bag?

(b) How many milligrams of furosemide will be preset in every 100 mL of the infusion fluid?

(c) If the patient only received 150 mL of the infusion, what amount of dextrose in grams was administered to the patient?

46. Approximately 2 L of 10% dextrose saline contains 80 mg of potassium chloride and was ordered to be administered over 6 hours. The patient's veins got infiltrated at 1 hour 25 mins, and the infusion had to be stopped.

(a) What volume of the infusion fluid was administered?

(b) Approximately what amount of potassium chloride will be remaining in the infusion bag?

(c) What amount of dextrose will be remaining in the infusion bag after the line was stopped?

47. You receive an order to administer a rehydration fluid to a patient for 6 hours at the drop rate of 25 drops per minute. What volume of the rehydration fluid will be received by the patient at the end of the 6 hours if the drop factor is 16 drops per milliliter?

48. A physician ordered 500 mg of an antibiotic to be mixed in 2 L of normal saline and infused into a patient over 12 hours. The drop factor of the administration set is 20 drops per milliliter.

(a) How many milliliters of the infusion fluid should the patient receive in 1 hour?

(b) How many milliliters of the fluid should the patient receive per minute?

(c) How many drops of the fluid should the patient receive per minute?

(d) What is the ratio strength of the antibiotic in the intravenous fluid?

(e) How many milligrams of the antibiotic are present in every milliliter of the infusion solution?

(f) What amount of the antibiotic (in micrograms) will be delivered by each drop of the infusion solution?

49. Patient was told that he will start his infusion by 6 a.m. The infusion is 500 mL normal saline that should be administered at the rate of 50 drops per minute. Patient is curious to know when the infusion will be over if he starts his infusion at exactly 6 a.m. What will be your likely answer? The drop factor of the infusion set is 15 (15 drops per milliliter).

50. A nurse practitioner ordered that a 1 L infusion of 10% dextrose saline containing 200 mg of an aminophylline be infused into an asthmatic patient. The patient only received 600 mL of the infusion when side effects of aminophylline became manifest and the infusion had to be stopped. What amount of aminophylline in milligrams did the patient receive?

★ Star Question ★

The physician ordered that all the contents of a 10 mL vial of aminophylline injection solution (25 mg/mL) be emptied into a 500 mL normal saline for infusion. The physician further directed that the infusion be set such that the patient should receive 1.2255 mg of aminophylline per minute until the infusion is all gone. At what rate must the infusion be set (in drops per minute) if the infusion set drop factor is 16 drops per milliliter?

Answers to Chapter 10
Practice Questions

1. 12.5 g dextrose
2. (a) 125 mL
   (b) 12.5 g dextrose
3. 187.5 mg antibiotics
4. (a) 100 mL
   (b) 0.909 mg
   (c) 54.545 mg morphine
5. (a) 60 g
   (b) 562.5 mL
   (c) 45 g
6. (a) 300 mg
   (b) 60 mL
7. Approx. 16 drops per min
8. 1,200 min (20 hours)
9. 1,104 mL
10. 50 g dextrose
11. (a) 4 mEq
    (b) 6.67 mEq
    (c) 138.9 mg dextrose
12. (a) 281.25 mg
    (b) 562.5
13. (a) 50 mL
    (b) 0.833 mL
    (c) Approx. 13 drops
14. (a) 500 mL
    (b) 40 mg
    (c) 1,200 mg antibiotics
15. (a) 50 g
    (b) 50 mg antibiotics
    (c) 2.88 hours (172.8 minutes)
16. (a) 160 mg
    (b) 48 mg
17. 937.5 mL
18. 40 drops per min

19. 300 mins (5 hours)
20. (a) 166.667 mL per hour
    (b) 2.778 mL per min
    (c) Approx. 56 drops per min
21. 9 g
22. 32.5 mg hydrocortisone
23. (a) 5 mL
    (b) 250 mg dextrose
    (c) 20 mg aminophylline
24. (a) 25 g
    (b) 1.6 mg KCl
    (c) 32 mg KCl
    (d) 6.25 g dextrose
25. (a) 40 mL
    (b) 37.04 mg
    (c) 2.25 g NaCl
26. (a) 6,818.18 mg
    (b) 2,272.73 mL
    (c) 614.53 mg
27. Approx. 33 drops per min
28. 540 mL
29. 250 g
30. Approx. 53 hours
31. (a) 25 g
    (b) 200 g
    (c) 500 mL
    (d) 4.17 mL
    (e) Approx. 67 drops per min
32. (a) 37.5 g dextrose
    (b) 15 mEq
33. (a) 100 g
    (b) 0.03%
    (c) 45 mg beta blocker
34. (a) 312.5 mL
    (b) 31.25 g dextrose
    (c) 62.5 mg morphine
35. (a) 1,750 mg

    (b) 1,050 mL solution

    (c) 8.54 mg

    (d) 21.95 g dextrose

36. (a) 960 mL

    (b) 1.297 million units

    (c) 54.05 g dextrose

37. (a) 0.708 mL per min

    (b) Approx. 11 drops per min

38. 360 mL

39. Approx. 11 hours afterwards

40. (a) 1,920 mg

    (b) 768 mL

    (c) 0.15% (d) 226.67 mg

41. 600 units

42. (a)166.67 mL

    (b) 2.78 mL

    (c) Approx. 56 drops

    (d) 1:8,000

    (e) 0.125 mg

    (f) 6.25 mcg

43. 30 g dextrose

44. (a) 2.5 mg

    (b) 1,000 mg

    (c) 212.5 mg

45. (a) 8 mL

    (b) 39.37 mg

    (c) 7.38 g

46. (a) 472.2 mL

    (b) 61.11 mg

    (c) 152.78 g

47. 562.5 mL

48. (a) 166.67 mL

    (b) 2.78 mL

    (c) Approx. 56 drops per min

    (d) 1:4,000

    (e) 0.25 mg

    (f) 12.5 mcg

49. 2.5 hours from 6 a.m. (8:30 a.m.)
50. 120 mg

Solution to Star Question

When the 10 mL of the aminophylline is added to the 500 mL normal saline, the entire volume becomes

$$10 \text{ mL} + 500 \text{ mL} = 510 \text{ mL}$$

Adding 10 mL of the aminophylline solution into the bag introduces certain amount of the active ingredient to the entire volume of 510 mL. We get that amount through proportion, bearing in mind that each milliliter of the aminophylline solution contains 25 mg of aminophylline active ingredient.

1 mL solution → 25 mg aminophylline

10 mL solution → u

$$u = \frac{25 \text{ mg aminophylline}}{1 \text{ mL solution}} \times \frac{10 \text{ mL solution}}{1}$$

= 250 mg aminophylline

Hence we can say that 510 mL of the infusion now contains 250 mg of aminophylline.

If the physician wants the patient to receive 1.2255 mg of aminophylline per minute, how many milliliters should that be, bearing in mind that 250 mg of aminophylline is in 510 mL?

250 mg aminophylline → 510 mL infusion solution

1.2255 mg aminophylline → u

$$u = \frac{510 \text{ mL infusion solution}}{250 \text{ mg aminophylline}} \times \frac{1.2255 \text{ mg aminophylline}}{1}$$

= 2.5 mL

Technically, for the patient to receive 1.2255 mg of aminophylline per minute, the patient must receive 2.5 mL of the infusion mixture per minute.

But what does the volume (2.5 mL) mean in terms of the number of drops?

The drop factor will guide us in this. The drop factor of 16 drops per milliliter means that a volume of 1 mL is equivalent to 16 drops from the infusion set.

$$1 \text{ mL} \rightarrow 16 \text{ drops}$$
$$2.5 \text{ mL} \rightarrow u$$

$$u = \frac{16 \text{ drops}}{1 \text{ mL}} \times \frac{2.5 \text{ mL}}{1}$$

$$= 40 \text{ drops}$$

So the infusion must be set at 40 drops per minute for the patient to receive 1.2255 mg of aminophylline per minute.

Appendix

Introduction to Basic Mathematics

1.1 Introduction

In everyday pharmaceutical calculation, accuracy is very essential to ensure each patient gets the right dose of medication prescribed. As you would be involved in this vital process, it is very important that your skills in basic math are good. The following sections in this chapter will help you review and develop these basic skills.

1.2 Objectives

At the end of this chapter, students should be able to do the following:

- Add, subtract, multiply, and divide whole numbers
- Add, subtract, multiply, and divide fractions
- Add, subtract, multiply, and divide decimal number
- Convert decimal numbers to fractions, fractions to decimals, and both to percentages
- Understand the basic concept of the Roman numerals
- Explain the 12-hour and 24-hour time system

1.3 Whole Numbers

The term *whole number* is typically used in mathematics. They represent all the digit figures used when we count. They are sometimes referred to as natural numbers or counting numbers. They comprise all the positive integers, including zero, but do not include the negative integers, fractions, decimals, or percentages. The whole numbers are 0, 1, 2, 3, 4, 5, 6, 7, 8, 9 . . . These numbers are the foundation on which many other number sets may be built.

There are four basic operations for whole numbers: addition (+), subtraction (−), multiplication (×), and division (÷). The following sections will illustrate how these operations work.

1.3.1 Adding and Subtracting Whole Numbers

Addition of Whole Numbers

The addition of whole numbers simply means combining numbers together to produce a total, which is also referred to as the sum of the numbers. To add whole numbers, you need to place them in a column according to their respective place values (units, tens, hundreds, thousands, etc.) such that they can be added correctly. The digits are then added beginning from the unit side. If the sum in a particular place value is more than ten, the unit is written down and the number of tens is carried over to the next column. Given below are some examples of how to add whole numbers.

Examples

1. 14 + 6 =

Adding numbers with one or two digits is pretty straightforward. In general, you can do it mentally or use your fingers.

$$14$$
$$\underline{+\ 6}$$
$$20$$

410

2. 120 + 60 =

$$120$$
$$\underline{+\ 60}$$
$$180$$

As the number digit increases, it becomes trickier. The first step is to arrange the whole numbers in a column according to their place values, as shown above. Start by adding the numbers in the rightmost column (i.e., $0 + 0 = 0$) and writing the answers down. Then add the second column ($2 + 6 = 8$) and finally the third column ($1 + 0 = 1$). So the answer is 180.

Note: Adding zero before a number never changes the number.

3. 35 +18 =

$$35$$
$$\underline{+18}$$
$$53$$

This equation is a bit different from the ones above in that, if you add the first column ($5 + 8 = 13$), the answer would be 13. It would be wrong to write this down; rather, only 3 is going to be written while 1 is carried over to the next column. So what you have to add in this column would be $3 + 1 + 1 = 5$, making the answer 53.

4. When preparing a solution, you are required to add 35 mL of alcohol to 50 mL of water. What would be the final volume of this preparation?

The solution to this is simply adding 35 to 50.

i.e.,

$$35$$
$$\underline{+50}$$
$$85$$

The total volume of the preparation is 85 mL.

5. What is the total authorized quantity for a prescription of 30 tablets of Lipitor 10 mg with 1 repeat?

In this case, the prescribed quantity of Lipitor is 30 tablets with 1 repeat. This simply means adding 30 to another 30.

i.e., 30+30 or 30

+30

60

The answer is 60 tablets.

Likewise, if the question is for 2 repeats, then you would have to add 30 twice to the original quantity of 30. In this case, it would be 30 + 30 + 30 = 90 tablets.

Subtracting Whole Numbers

Subtraction of whole numbers is the opposite of addition; rather than adding two numbers to get a sum, one is removed from another to determine the difference. Similar to the addition process of whole numbers, when subtracting one whole number from another, we also line them up. Then we commence subtracting each number separately, starting from the right and moving towards the left.

Examples

1. 7 – 2 =

To carry out this task, align the digits as shown below and then subtract. Subtraction simple means taking away. So you would be taking away 2 from 7, as shown below.

7

– 2

5

2.   15 – 5 =

Likewise, regroup as below and take away 5 from 5; that gives 0. Then take away 0 from 1, which would be 1.

$$15$$
$$\underline{-\ 5}$$
$$10$$

3.   378 – 253 =

$$378$$
$$\underline{-253}$$
$$125$$

4.   The cost of a prescription of EpiPen is $75. If the customer gives you a $100 bill for payment, how much change would you give the customer?

This question requires you to subtract $75 from $100.

i.e.,

$$100$$
$$\underline{-\ 75}$$
$$25$$

The change for the customer is $25.

5.   The stock bottle of metformin contains 500 tablets. If the pharmacist dispensed 360 tablets to a patient, how many tablets of metformin are remaining in the stock container?

Similarly, subtracting 360 from 500 would give the amount of tablets remaining in the container.

i.e.,

$$
\begin{array}{r}
500 \\
- 360 \\
\hline
140
\end{array}
$$

1.3.2 Multiplying and Dividing Whole numbers

Multiplying Whole Numbers

The best way to describe multiplication of whole numbers is repeated addition. For instance, multiplying 2 × 3 is the same as adding 2 + 2 + 2; likewise, 2 × 4 = 2 + 2 + 2 + 2. For easier calculation, it is better for the multiplier to be the one with less value, i.e., 3 × 2 = 3 + 3 and 4 × 2 = 4 + 4. Whichever way it is done, the final result is not affected. The symbol '×' denotes "multiplication" or "times." The numbers in a product are called factors. For example, 7 × 3 = 21; in this example, 7 and 3 are factors of the product 21. When we multiply whole numbers, we need to line up the numbers correctly, just as we did with addition and subtraction of whole numbers.

Examples

1. 5 × 3 =

i.e., 5 + 5 + 5 = 15 or

$$
\begin{array}{r}
5 \\
\times 3 \\
\hline
15
\end{array}
$$

2. $43 \times 6 =$

This requires multiplying all the top figures by just the bottom one.

$$
\begin{array}{r}
43 \\
\times\,6 \\
\hline
258
\end{array}
$$

The first step is to multiply 6 in the second row by 3 in the first row, i.e., $3 \times 6 = 18$. Then write 8 and save 1. The next step is to multiply 6 again with 4 from the top row (i.e., $4 \times 6 = 24$). Then add the 1 saved earlier to this value. This becomes $24 + 1 = 25$. Write this down so the product or answer is 258.

3. $136 \times 15 =$

Again, the first step is aligning the numbers, as shown below. Then, using 5 from the bottom row, multiply each of the figures in the upper row and write the results down. After completing that, the same process is repeated with 1 from the bottom row with all the numbers in the upper row. The answer is written as shown below. Be sure to keep the alignment correct. The rows for the answers are then added to give the final product.

$$
\begin{array}{r}
136 \\
\times\,15 \\
\hline
680 \\
+136 \\
\hline
2{,}040
\end{array}
$$

4. The direction for a prescription of 500 mg cephalexin requires that a patient takes one tablet 4 times a day. If the patient is to take the medication for 10 days, how many tablets of cephalexin are needed?

This problem is a direct multiplication of 10 and 4,

i.e.,

$$
\begin{array}{r}
10 \\
\times\,4 \\
\hline
40 \text{ tablets}
\end{array}
$$

5. The record of a patient states that 33 boxes of Victoza were dispensed last year. If each box of Victoza is 6 mL, what is the total volume of Victoza in milliliters dispensed last year to the patient?

$$
\begin{array}{r}
33 \\
\times\,6 \\
\hline
198 \text{ mL}
\end{array}
$$

Dividing Whole Numbers

Division is the process by which we try to find out how many times a number is contained in another number. Essentially, it is the opposite operation of multiplication; therefore, we can use multiplication to verify the accuracy of division. It is represented by the symbol ÷. The number being divided is called the dividend, while the other number use to divide is called the divisor. The result of the operation is known as the quotient (dividend / *divisor* = quotient).

Examples

1.   45 ÷ 5 = 9

In this case, 5 is the divisor, 45 is the dividend, and 9 is the quotient. Normally, in division operation, the divisor is usually less than the dividend. In this example, 5 is contained in 45 nine times (i.e., 5 × 9 = 45).

As the value of the dividend increases, it becomes more difficult to calculate. To simplify the process, we can make use of long division.

2.   720 ÷ 8 = 90

$$
\begin{array}{r}
90 \\
8)\,\overline{720} \\
-\ \underline{72} \\
0
\end{array}
$$

Normally, the first step is to divide 7 by 8. As this will not yield a whole number because 7 is smaller than 8, we proceed to 72, which can be divided by 8. In this case, 72 could be divided into 8 nine times. Finally, 8 into zero will be zero. Hence, the answer to the question is 90.

3.   540 ÷ 30 = 18

As 5 cannot be divided by 30, move 5 and 4 to be 54. Now, 54 can be divided into 30 one time with a remainder of 24. So we write 1 at the answer position and proceed to joining 24 and the 0, making 240. What we have left is 240 ÷ 30. At this point, the zeros in 240 and 30 can actually cancel out, making it just 24 ÷ 3. This becomes easy; 24 can divide into 3 eight times. So you write this beside the 1 in the answer position to make the final answer, which is 18.

This is another way to look at this:

$$
\frac{540}{30} = \frac{54}{3} \text{ (when zeros cancel out)} = 18
$$

4. $360 \div 12 = 30$

$$
\begin{array}{r}
30 \\
12\overline{)360} \\
\underline{36} \\
00
\end{array}
$$

Similarly, 36 divided by 12 is 3, and 0 divided by 12 is zero. The answer is 30.

5. You received a new prescription to dispense a total of 450 mg of ramipril capsule. If you are to use the 5 mg capsule, how many capsules of ramipril would you dispense to the patient?

This question requires dividing 450 by 5, i.e.,

$$450 \div 5$$

Again, as 4 cannot be divided by 5 to yield a whole number, move both numbers together. This means dividing 45 into 5. This gives 9. Then we divide 0 by 5, which is zero. Therefore, $450 \div 5 = 90$.

Total number of capsules required is 90.

1.4 Fractions

A fraction represents parts of a whole number, and it's usually written in forms like $\frac{3}{4}, \frac{1}{2}, \frac{1}{4}$, and so on. The upper or first figure is referred to as the *numerator*, and it indicates how many parts of the whole there are. The lower or second figure on the other hand is called the *denominator*, and it tells us how many parts are in the whole. Thus, in the fraction $\frac{3}{4}$, 3 is the numerator and 4 is the denominator.

Where the numerator is less than the denominator, it's known as a *proper fraction*, and the result is less than 1. For example, $\frac{1}{4}$ is considered a proper fraction because the denominator (4) is greater than the numerator (1). On the other hand, if the numerator is greater than the denominator, it is called an *improper fraction*, and the result is always greater than 1. For instance, in the fraction $\frac{5}{2}$, the numerator (5) is greater than the denominator (2), so it is an improper fraction. A fraction can also be a *mixed fraction*; in this case, it would contain both whole numbers and proper fractions (e.g., $2\frac{2}{3}$, $5\frac{1}{4}$). The value of the fraction resulting from dividing the fraction is the *quotient*.

1.4.1 Addition and Subtraction of Fraction

The first step in adding or subtracting a fraction is to reduce them to a common denomination; that is, having the same numeral and then adding the numerator without altering the denominator. If the denominator is the same, we would retain it as the common denominator. Then the value of dividing this by each of the denominator is multiplied by the numerator. The numerator can then be added and the result reduced if possible. Consider the following examples.

Examples

1. $\frac{4}{7} + \frac{2}{7} =$

Both fractions have the same denominator, thus the common denominator is 7.

$$\text{Hence, } \frac{4+2}{7} = \frac{6}{7}$$

Therefore, the answer is $\frac{6}{7}$.

2. $\frac{2}{4} + \frac{1}{3} =$

Since the denominators are different in this case, we have to determine the lowest common denominator (LCD), i.e., the smallest whole number that can be divided equally by both denominators 4 and 3.

This is 12. Therefore, the equivalent for both of these fractions would be $\dfrac{6}{12} + \dfrac{4}{12}$.

$$\text{Thus, } \frac{6+4}{12} = \frac{10}{12-} = \frac{5}{6}$$

The answer is $\dfrac{10}{12}$. This can further be reduced to $\dfrac{5}{6}$ as the answer (by dividing both 10 and 12 by the same number—2).

3. $\dfrac{5}{7} + \dfrac{3}{4} =$

The lowest common denominator that would divide both denominators evenly in this case is 28. Hence, the resulting equivalent fractions: $\dfrac{20}{28} + \dfrac{21}{28}$.

$$\frac{20+21}{28} = \frac{41}{28} = 1\frac{13}{28}$$

The answer is an improper fraction and can further be reduced to $1\dfrac{13}{28}$.

4. $1\dfrac{2}{3} + \dfrac{3}{5} =$

Because $1\dfrac{2}{3}$ is a mixed fraction, the first step is to convert it to an improper fraction. This is done by multiplying 3 by 1 and adding 2, which is equal to $\dfrac{5}{3}$. So we can rewrite the equation as $\dfrac{5}{3} + \dfrac{3}{5}$.

LCD is 15, thus

$$\frac{25+9}{15} = \frac{34}{15}$$

Similarly, the answer can be reduced to $2\dfrac{4}{15}$.

5. When compounding an ointment for a patient, the pharmacist used $\frac{2}{10}$ of a specific medication on the first day. The technician also used $\frac{3}{10}$ of the original quantity of same medication the next day to make similar preparation. What fraction of the medication has been used up?

The question requires adding the two fractions together. If we write the equation out, it will be $\frac{2}{10} + \frac{3}{10}$.

$$\frac{2+3}{10} = \frac{5}{10} = \frac{1}{2}$$

6. $\frac{4}{7} - \frac{3}{7} =$

In the above equation, do not make the mistake of just subtracting the figures directly. The LCD is still needed to complete the operation; the same rule applies as in addition. As the denominators are the same, the LCD does not change; therefore, it's 7 (i.e., $7 \div 7 = 1$, $1 \times 4 = 4$, and $1 \times 3 = 3$). Thus,

$$\frac{4-3}{7} = \frac{1}{7}$$

7. $\frac{1}{2} - \frac{3}{8} =$

When the denominators are different, the LCD of both numbers needs to be determined, just as in the case with addition. In this case, 8 is actually divisible by both numbers; therefore, it is an appropriate LCD.

Hence, $8 \div 2 = 4$; $4 \times 1 = 4$.
Also, $8 \div 8 = 1$; $1 \times 3 = 3$.

Thus,

$$\frac{4-3}{8} = \frac{1}{8}$$

8. $\dfrac{4}{5} - \dfrac{1}{3} =$

LCD of the denominators is 15.

Hence, $15 \div 5 = 3$; $3 \times 4 = 12$ and $15 \div 3 = 5$; $5 \times 1 = 5$.

The equation becomes

$$\frac{12-5}{15} = \frac{7}{15}$$

9. $\dfrac{28}{6} - \dfrac{14}{6} =$

LCD is 6, so the equation can be written as,

$$\frac{28}{6} - \frac{14}{6} = \frac{14}{6}$$

10. If at the start of your shift at the pharmacy you have $\dfrac{5}{6}$ gallon of distilled water and at the end of the day the quantity remaining is just $\dfrac{2}{8}$ gallon of the original quantity. What fraction of distilled water has been used up?

The equation here is,

$$\frac{5}{6} - \frac{2}{8} =$$

The LCD is 24, so we can rewrite the equation as,

$$\frac{20-6}{24} = \frac{14}{24} \text{ or } \frac{7}{12}$$

1.4.2 Multiplication and Division of Fraction

Unlike addition and subtraction of fractions, multiplication of fractions is easier and straightforward. No LCD is required; direct multiplying of the numerators and the denominators will do. The results are normally reduced to its lowest fraction. Also, if the numbers of the numerator and denominator can be divided by a common number, the equation can be further simplified by reducing it to the smallest indivisible fraction before multiplying. Furthermore, when mixed fractions are involved, it must be converted to an improper fraction before the operation can be carried out.

Similarly, when dividing fractions, most of these rules apply; for mixed fractions, change it to improper fractions. After which is the reciprocal or reversal of the divisor, making the denominator become the nominator and vice versa. Then direct multiplication of the numbers in the fractions. Again, it is always appropriate to simplify the results by reducing to the smallest indivisible fraction where possible. This can be done by dividing both numerator and denominator by a common factor that can divide both without any remainder.

Examples

1. $\dfrac{2}{6} \times \dfrac{3}{4} =$

First, multiply the numerator and denominator directly, and then simplify the results. Thus,

$$\frac{2 \times 3}{6 \times 4} = \frac{6}{24} = \frac{1}{4}$$

2. $\dfrac{6}{8} \times \dfrac{7}{8} =$

Similarly,

$$\frac{6 \times 7}{8 \times 8} = \frac{42}{64} = \frac{21}{32}$$

3. $\dfrac{16 \times 2}{7 \times 3} =$ $\qquad$ $\dfrac{16 \times 2}{7 \times 3} = \dfrac{32}{21} = 1\dfrac{11}{21}$

4. $4\dfrac{3}{4} \times 5\dfrac{3}{4} =$ $\qquad$ $\dfrac{19}{4} \times \dfrac{23}{4} = \dfrac{19 \times 23}{4 \times 4} = \dfrac{437}{16} = 27\dfrac{5}{16}$

5. $\dfrac{5}{6} \div \dfrac{6}{10} =$ 　　　　$\dfrac{5}{6} \times \dfrac{10}{6} = \dfrac{50}{36} = \dfrac{25}{18} = 1\dfrac{7}{18}$

6. $\dfrac{11}{2} \div \dfrac{1}{4} =$ 　　　　$\dfrac{11}{2} \times \dfrac{4}{1} = \dfrac{44}{2} = 22$

7. $\dfrac{3}{4} \div \dfrac{1}{2} =$ 　　　　$\dfrac{3 \times 2}{4 \times 1} = \dfrac{6}{4} = \dfrac{3}{2} = 1\dfrac{1}{2}$

8. $\dfrac{9}{10} \div \dfrac{4}{3} = \dfrac{9 \times 3}{10 \times 4} = \dfrac{27}{40}$

1.5 Decimal

Decimals are another way of writing fractions. They can actually be viewed as fractions with denominators of power of 10 (10, 100, 1000, etc). However, the denominator is never written because the decimal point indicates the place values of the numerals to a fraction or even to a percentage.

Examples of decimals are 0.1 (which is same as $\dfrac{1}{10}$), 0.01 (or $\dfrac{1}{100}$), and 0.45 (or $\dfrac{45}{100}$). To convert a fraction to a decimal, the numerator is divided by the denominator. For instance, to convert the fraction $\dfrac{3}{4}$ to a decimal, we would rewrite the equation as shown below and then carry out the division.

$$3 \div 4 = 0.75 \text{ Therefore, } \dfrac{3}{4} = 0.75$$

Similarly, $\dfrac{1}{4}$ can be converted to a decimal as follows:

$$1 \div 4 = 0.25 \qquad \text{Thus, } \dfrac{1}{4} = 0.25$$

Also, $\dfrac{2}{5} = 2 \div 5 = 0.4$

In the same way, a decimal can easily be changed to a fraction. To do this, the decimal number is the numerator of the fraction while the denominator is considered to be 1 with 0s equal to the number of decimal places. For instance, consider the last example above. We could convert 0.4 to a fraction by making 4 the numerator and set the denominator to 10 because there is only one place after the decimal.

$$\text{Therefore, } 0.4 = \frac{4}{10}$$

This can further be reduced by dividing both numerator and denominator by 2.

$$\text{Hence, } \frac{4}{10} = \frac{2}{5}$$

Also, 0.75 can be converted to a fraction as follows:

$$0.75 = \frac{75}{100} \qquad \text{This can be reduced to } \frac{3}{4}$$

$$\text{Likewise, } 0.125 = \frac{125}{1,000} = \frac{1}{8}$$

1.5.1 Rounding of Decimals

To avoid errors in the pharmacy, decimals are always preceded by a trailing zero, e.g., 0.15 mL, 0.30 g, 0.125 mcg. This helps prevent confusion and minimize errors in doses. Also, to help make measurement easy or where accurate calculation of a dose is needed, decimals are rounded up to a small number of decimal places. This is done such that the whole number on the left of the decimal is not affected, only the figures after it. To round up a number, it must be equal or more than 5. In this case, the number is dropped and 1 is added to the rounding digit. If a number is less than 5, no further action is needed, and the entire digit to the right is ignored to meet up with the desired number of decimal places. For instance, 7.3 can be rounded up to just 7, while 7.6 can be rounded up to 8.

However, because of the level of accuracy needed in dosing, rounding numbers might not be applicable in all situations. But sometimes it is acceptable to do so. For example, if the calculated dose for a child is 5.95 mL of amoxicillin suspension, because it can be difficult to accurately measure this dose at home, rounding this up to 6 mL would seem more appropriate.

1.5.2 Addition and Subtraction of Decimals

All operations with decimal numbers are carried out in a similar manner as with whole numbers. However, it is important to position the decimal point appropriately to avoid error. After aligning the digits properly, we would add or subtract, as in the case of whole numbers.

Examples

1.   6.25 + 5.85

Write the digits in vertical columns, align them, and add as below:

$$
\begin{array}{r}
6.25 \\
+\ 5.85 \\
\hline
12.10
\end{array}
$$

2.   13.145 + 8.98 =

$$
\begin{array}{r}
13.145 \\
+\ 8.980 \\
\hline
22.125
\end{array}
$$

3.   0.215 + 3.175 =

$$
\begin{array}{r}
0.215 \\
+\ 3.175 \\
\hline
3.390
\end{array}
$$

4. 4.97 – 2.33 =

$$
\begin{array}{r}
4.97 \\
-\ 2.33 \\
\hline
2.64
\end{array}
$$

5. 44.673 –12.435 =

$$
\begin{array}{r}
44.673 \\
-\ 12.435 \\
\hline
32.238
\end{array}
$$

6. 0.982 – 0.75 =

$$
\begin{array}{r}
0.982 \\
-\ 0.750 \\
\hline
0.232
\end{array}
$$

1.5.3 Multiplication and Division of Decimals

Multiplying Decimals

The process for multiplying a decimal is similar to that of whole numbers. Unlike with addition and subtraction of fractions, the alignment of decimal places is not necessary during the operation; however, proper positioning of it is required at the end of the calculation. Any zero after the decimal may be removed; this would have no effect on its value and makes the multiplication easier.

Examples

1. 0.25 × 0.2 =

First, multiply normally, ignoring the decimal, then place the decimal by counting back the combined decimal places of the original numbers. In this case, it is 3.

Thus,

$$0.25$$
$$\times \underline{0.2}$$
$$050$$
$$+\underline{000}$$
$$0050$$

So counting 3 decimal places back,

$$= 0.050 \text{ (or 0.05)}$$

2. $10.20 \times 1.1 =$

Similarly, multiply directly without considering the decimals. This equation can be simplified by ignoring the zero after decimals.

Thus,

$$10.2$$
$$\times \underline{1.1}$$
$$102$$
$$+\underline{102}$$
$$1,122$$

$$= 11.22 \text{ (Since the number of decimal places is 2)}$$

3. $45.13 \times 1.5 =$

$$\text{Thus: } 45.13$$
$$\times \underline{1.5}$$
$$22,565$$
$$+\underline{4,513}$$
$$67,695 = 67.695 \text{ (Number of}$$
$$\text{decimal places 3)}$$

4.   810.25 × 10 =

In this case, the multiplier is 10; this makes it easy to calculate. If the multiplier is a multiple of 10, rather than going through the whole process of multiplication, the decimal can be moved to the right according to the number of zeros in the multiplier, and this gives us the answer. In the above equation, the number of zeros in the multiplier (10) is one. So we just move the number of decimals to the right by one place.

Hence, 810.25 × 10 = 8,102.5

5.   0.0056 × 1,000 =

Here there are three zeros in the multiplier (1,000).
Therefore, 0.0056 × 1,000 = 5.6

Dividing Decimals

When dividing decimals, the approach is very similar to dividing whole numbers. It is easier when the numbers we are dividing are changed to whole numbers. This is done by shifting the decimal point of both numbers to the right (i.e., the divisor and the dividend).

6.   6.4 ÷ 0.4 =

First, we need to change the divisor to a whole number by shifting both decimals to the right. Therefore, $\frac{6.4}{0.4} = \frac{64}{4}$ = 16. (Carry out the normal long division process)

7.   5.25 ÷ 1.2 =

Similarly, this equation is the same as 52.5 ÷ 12 = $\frac{52.5}{12}$ = 4.375

8. $1.44 \div 0.6 =$

$$14.4 \div 6 = \frac{14.4}{6} = 2.4$$

9. $2.52 \div 0.51 =$

$$252 \div 51 = \frac{252}{51} = 4.94$$

10. $12.40 \div 62 =$

In this case, 62 cannot be divided into 12.4. We can therefore ignore the decimal place (one decimal place) for now, but remember to apply it at the end of the calculation. Hence, we can carry out this task as follows:

$$\frac{124}{62} = 2 = 0.2 \text{ (apply one decimal place)}$$

1.6 Percentages

The term *percent* means an expression in parts of a hundred. It's usually denoted as %. For instance, 20% means 20 parts in each one hundred of the same portion. Fractions can easily be converted to percentages by dividing the numerator by the denominator then multiplying by 100. Likewise, a decimal is converted to percentage via multiplying by 100, which simply means moving the decimal places forward. Similarly, percentages can easily be converted to fractions or decimals by dividing it by 100.

Examples

Convert the following fractions to percent

1. $\dfrac{3}{8}$

$$\frac{3}{8} \times 100 = 37.5\%$$

2. $\dfrac{3}{4}$

$$\dfrac{3}{4} \times 100 = 75\%$$

3. $\dfrac{1}{2}$

$$\dfrac{1}{2} \times 100 = 50\%$$

Convert the following percent to fraction

4. 60%

$$\dfrac{60}{100} = \dfrac{6}{10} = \dfrac{3}{5}$$

5. 16%

$$\dfrac{16}{100} = \dfrac{4}{25}$$

6. 5%

$$\dfrac{5}{100} = \dfrac{1}{20}$$

Convert the following decimals to percentages

7. 0.5

$$0.5 \times 100 = 50\%$$

8. 0.02

$$0.02 \times 100 = 2\%$$

9. 0.0125

$$0.0125 \times 100 = 1.25\%$$

Convert the following percentages to decimals

10. 5%

$$\frac{5}{100} = 0.05$$

11. 75%

$$\frac{75}{100} = 0.75$$

12. 11% =

$$\frac{11}{100} = 0.11$$

1.7 Roman Numerals

The Roman numeral is a system of numbering used in ancient Rome whereby alphabetical letters are used to represent numbers. It utilizes a few letters of the alphabet in a logical pattern to express numbers. Occasionally, Roman numerals are used in prescriptions to express quantities.

There are eight letters of standard values that are employed, and others are gotten by combining, adding to, or subtracting from them. These are the letters:

I or i = 1; V or v = 5; X or x = 10;

L or l = 50; C or c = 100; D or d = 500;

and M or m = 1,000.

The numbers one to ten are written I, II, III, IV, V, VI, VII, VIII, IX, and X. Other quantities are formed by combining letters. There is no letter for the value zero, and half $(\frac{1}{2})$ is represented as ss. The general rules in expressing quantities are as follows:

1. When a letter is repeated, it means its value should be repeated. For instance, if x =10, xx would be 10 + 10 = 20.
2. Letters placed after a letter of greater value would add to the value of that number. For example, vii (5+2) = 7 or xi (10 +1) = 11
3. Similarly, a letter placed before would reduce its quantity by the value. E.g., iv (5 – 1) = 4 or ix (10 – 1) = 9.
4. Finally, once there is a bar above a letter or group of letters, it increases its value by a thousand.

Examples

ix = 9	xix = 19	xl = 40
xiii = 13	xxi = 21	l = 50
xiv = 14	xxv = 25	lx = 60
xviii = 18	xxx = 30	lxxi = 71

1.8 The 12-Hour and 24-Hour Timing System

Time is generally presented in the 12-hour system. In this case, it runs from midnight to midday and then repeats the cycle. To differential this time, the periods from midnight to noon (morning period) are represented with AM (e.g., 1 a.m., 2 a.m., etc.) while the periods from noon to midnight (evening period) are represented with PM (e.g., 1 p.m., 2 p.m., etc.). AM and PM are Latin words and stand for *ante meridiem* and *post meridiem*, which means "*before noon*" and "*after noon*" respectively.

However, sometimes the 24-hour timing system is also utilized to describe time. The 24-hour timing system is a standard of reporting time whereby the whole day is divided into twenty-four hours and starts from midnight. As the time runs from zero to twenty-three, there is no repeat and need to differentiate between the morning and evening period. The time in this case is represented as 01:00 hrs, 02:00 hrs, and so on.

In general, the 24-hour time system has been popular for many years. It has been widely employed in various areas and has been used by the military, scientists, navigators, and so on. In the pharmacy practice, the 24-hour system is sometimes used when writing a prescription to specify time because it helps prevent error due to vagueness.

The table below illustrates the conversion between the 12- and 24-hour system. When converting to the 24-hour system, add 12 to the PM hours, starting from 1 p.m. to midnight, e.g., 2 p.m. = 1400 hours (hrs). No action is required for hours from 1a.m. to noon and between 12:01 p.m. to 12:59 p.m., as the time would still be the same, i.e., 10 a.m. = 1000 hrs. However, between midnight and 12:59 a.m., subtract 12 to get the time, e.g. 12:30 a.m. is 00:30 min (12.30 – 12 = 0.30).

Similarly, to change from the 24-hour system to AM and PM, subtract 12 hours from time between 1300 hrs to 000 and add PM. From 1200 hrs to 1259 hrs, just add PM, e.g., 12:40 is 12:40 p.m., and from 01:00 to 11:59 hrs, just add the AM, e.g., 03:00 hrs is 3:00 a.m. Finally, from midnight to 00:59, add 12 hours and AM after the time, so 00:39 hrs will be 12:39 a.m.

Time Systems

12 hrs	1 a.m.	3 a.m.	7 a.m.	11 a.m.	12 p.m.	2 p.m.	6 p.m.	8 p.m.	12 a.m.
24 hrs	01:00	03:00	07:00	11:00	12:00	14:00	18:00	20:00	00:00

Appendix Practice Questions

1. 32 mg + 18 mg =

2. 120 mL – 60 mL =

3. 100 × 521 kg =

4. 3,500 mL × 120 =

5. 1,200 mg ÷ 100 =

6. 120 units ÷ 4 =

7. $ 10.25 + $13.43 + $11.45 =

8. 480.50 g – 120.68 g =

9. 9.82 +16.90 + 0.456 =

10. 180 mL – 22.16 mL =

11. 0.37 × 0.25 =

12. 1.5 ÷ 0.3 =

13. 41.623 × 1.23 =

14. 0.250 x 0.100 =

15. 0.72 x 0.8 =

16. $\frac{4}{9} + \frac{5}{9} =$

17. $\frac{1}{5} + \frac{9}{10} =$

18. $\frac{8}{7} - \frac{1}{3} =$

19. $\frac{18}{4} - \frac{3}{2} =$

20. $\frac{4}{7} \times \frac{3}{11} =$

21. $3\frac{1}{2} \times \frac{3}{4} =$

22. $\frac{3}{5} \div \frac{8}{10} =$

23. $4\frac{1}{2}$ tsp $\div 1\frac{3}{4}$ tsp =

24. Convert the following to decimal:

a) $\frac{15}{9}$ b) $3\frac{5}{8}$ c) $6\frac{3}{5}$

25. Convert the following to fractions:
    a) 0.65   b) 0.450   c) 0. 625

26. Convert the following fractions to percent:
    a) $\frac{2}{5}$ b) $\frac{12}{13}$ c) $\frac{18}{60}$

27. Convert the following percentages to fractions:
    a) 15%   b) 45%   c) 5%

28. Convert the following decimals to percentage:
    a) 0.03   b) 0.73   c) 0.2

29. Round 9.332 to the nearest whole number.

30. Write the following in Roman numeral:
    a) 17   b) 23   c) 38

31. Convert to digital numbers.
    a) viii   b) xxii   c) xxv

32. When compounding a drug in the pharmacy, a pharmacy assistant weighed out 28.80 g of a diclofenac powder and mixed it up with 451.20 g of Diffusimax gel. What is the total weight of the final product?

33. A patient has 360 capsules of ramipril 10 mg on file and asked you to fill 90 capsules. After filling his prescription, how many more ramipril 10 mg capsules are remaining on file for the patient?

34. In preparing dexamethasone syrup, a pharmacy technician requires 8 mL of simple syrup for each preparation. If the total amount of simple syrup available at the pharmacy is 64 mL, how many dexamethasone preparations can be made from this volume of syrup?

35. A patient's dose for Lantus insulin is 40 units per day. How many units does the patient require in 30 days?

36. Each box of Humalog insulin contains 1,500 units. If John uses 15 units every day, how many days would this last for?

37. The cost of a prescription is $30 for every pack of Ensure liquid. If the patient needs 15 packs, what would his total cost for these packs be?

38. The weight of cyclobenzaprine powder in each topical ointment preparation is 3.5 mg. If the total number of preparation at the end is 9, what is the total amount of cyclobenzaprine powder used in all the preparations?

39. While dispensing in the pharmacy, only $\frac{2}{3}$ of the original clindamycin powder was remaining at the end of the day. What fraction of the original powder was used?

40. If there are only $5\frac{1}{2}$ lb of Diclofenac powder remaining and the pharmacy uses $\frac{3}{4}$ lb daily, how long will this stock last?

41. The dose of amoxicillin suspension for a child is $5\frac{3}{4}$ teaspoons per day. How many milliliters would the child require for ten days? (1 tsp = 5 mL)

42. Each metformin stock bottle contains 1,000 tablets when full. If at the end of the day $2\frac{3}{4}$ bottles were used up, how many tablets were dispensed that day?

43. The quantity of prednisolone liquid at hand was 109.70 mL. If the pharmacist dispensed 25.5 mL to a patient, how much prednisolone would be left?

44. In preparing a topical ointment for a patient, the pharmacy technician weighed out and compounded the following ingredients: diltiazem powder, 4.85 g, and Vaseline, 58.8 g. What is the total weight of the ointment?

45. A customer presented a $50 bill to pay for his prescriptions. If the costs of his prescriptions are Lantus ($15.28), Victoza ($12.15), and metformin ($8.26), how much change do you owe him?

46. The instruction on the label of azithromycin suspension for a child states that 5.25 mL of the suspension should be taken on the first day and then 2.63 mL each day for four days. What is the volume of azithromycin required for this child?

47. A patient takes 12.5 mg of methotrexate daily. If each tablet contains 2.5 mg of methotrexate, how many tablets is the patient taking per day?

48. The dose of cephalexin suspension for a nine-month-old child is 2.5 mL to be taken four times a day. What is the child's total daily dose in milliliters?

49. The prescription for a patient states this: Take 1.9 mL of fluoxetine liquid once daily for fourteen days. How much fluoxetine in milliliters would you dispense for this patient?

50. State the time in the12-hour system for these prescriptions:
    a) Nitroglycerine patches 0.2 mg/hr. Apply daily at 0800 hrs and remove at 2000 hrs.
    b) Levetiracetam 250 mg at 1300 hrs and 500 mg at 2200 hrs.

Answers to Appendix Practice Questions

1. 50 mg

2. 60 mL

3. 52,100 kg

4. 420,000 mL

5. 12 mg

6. 30 units

7. $35.13

8. 359.82 g

9. 27.176

10. 157.84 mL

11. 0.0925

12. 5

13. 51.20

14. 0.025

15. 0.576

16. 1

17. $1\frac{1}{10}$

18. $\frac{17}{21}$

19. 3

20. $\frac{12}{77}$

21. $\frac{21}{8}$ or $2\frac{5}{8}$

22. $\frac{3}{4}$

23. $2\frac{4}{7}$ tsp

24. a) 1.67

    b) 3.63

    c) 6.6

25. a) $\frac{13}{20}$

    b) $\frac{9}{20}$

    c) $\frac{5}{8}$

26. a) 40%

    b) 92%

    c) 30%

27. a) $\frac{3}{20}$

    b) $\frac{9}{20}$

    c) $\frac{1}{20}$

28. a) 3%

    b) 73%

    c) 20%

29. 9

30. a) XVII

    b) XXIII

    c) XXXVIII

31. a) 8

    b) 22

    c) 25

32. 480 g

33. 270 capsules

34. 8

35. 1,200 units

36. 100 days

37. $450

38. 31.5 mg

39. $\frac{1}{3}$

40. 7 days

41. 287.5 mL

42. 2,750

43. 84.20 mL

44. 63,65 g

45. $14.31

46. 15.77 mL

47. 5 tablets

48. 10 mL

49. 26.6 mL

50. a) 8.00 a.m. and 8.00 p.m.

   b) 1.00 p.m. and 10.00 p.m.

BIBLIOGRAPHY

Alberta College of Pharmacists: *"Standards of Practice"* (Last revised May 2014)

Allen, L. V. (Jnr), Popovich, N. G., Ansel, H. C: *Pharmaceutical dosage forms and drug delivery systems*, 9th Edition, Baltimore, 2011, Lippincott Williams & Wilkins.

Ansel, H.C., Stoklosa, M. J: *Pharmaceutical Calculations*, 12th Edition, Baltimore, 2006, Lippincott Williams &Wilkins.

Fulcher, R. M., Fulcher, E. M: *Math Calculations for Pharmacy technicians A work text,* 2nd Edition, Missouri, 2013, Elsevier.

Neumiller,J.J., Steelman, B., Davis, K., Beale,E., Mizner,J.J., Beccarelli, J: *Pharmacy Technician Principles and Practice*, 4th Edition, Missouri, 2016,Elsevier.

Shargel, L.,Mutnik, A. H., Souney, P. F., Swanson, L.N: *Comprehensive Pharmacy Review,* 7th Edition, Baltimore, 2010, Lippincott Williams &Wilkins.

Thompson, J. T: *A Practical Guide to Contemporary Pharmacy Practice*, 3rd Edition, Baltimore, 2009, Lippincott Williams &Wilkins.

INDEX

www.ingramcontent.com/pod-product-compliance
Lightning Source LLC
Chambersburg PA
CBHW020720180526
45163CB00001B/43